Bates' Pocket Guide to

Physical Examination and History Taking

FOURTH EDITION

Bates' Pocket Guide to

Physical Examination and History Taking

Lynn S. Bickley, MD
*Associate Professor of Internal Medicine
and Neuropsychiatry
Departments of Internal Medicine and Neuropsychiatry
Associate Dean for Curriculum
Texas Tech University Health Sciences Center
Lubbock, Texas*

Peter G. Szilagyi, MD, MPH
*Professor of Pediatrics
Chief, Division of General Pediatrics
University of Rochester School of Medicine and Dentistry
Rochester, New York*

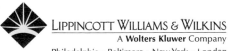

LIPPINCOTT WILLIAMS & WILKINS
A **Wolters Kluwer** Company

Philadelphia • Baltimore • New York • London
Buenos Aires • Hong Kong • Sydney • Tokyo

Senior Acquisitions Editor: Elizabeth Nieginski
Senior Development Editor: Renee Gagliardi
Editorial Assistant: Joshua Levandoski
Senior Production Editor: Sandra Cherrey Scheinin
Senior Production Manager: Helen Ewan
Managing Editor / Production: Erika Kors
Art Director: Carolyn O'Brien
Designer: Melissa Olson
Illustration Coordinator: Brett MacNaughton
Manufacturing Manager: William Alberti
Indexer: Katherine Pitcoff
Compositor: Circle Graphics
Printer: R. R. Donnelley & Sons Company/Crawfordsville

4th Edition

9 8 7 6 5 4 3

Library of Congress Cataloging-in-Publication Data
Bickley, Lynn S.
    Bates' pocket guide to physical examination and history taking / Lynn S. Bickley, Peter G. Szilagyi.—4th ed.
        p. ; cm.
    Includes index.
    ISBN 0-7817-3818-0 (alk. paper)
        1. Physical diagnosis I. Title: Pocket guide to physical examination and history taking.
    II. Szilagyi, Peter G. III. Bates, Barbara, 1928- IV. Title.
        [DNLM: 1. Medical History Taking—Handbooks. 2. Physical Examination—methods—Handbooks. WB 39 B583b 2004]
    RC76.B38 2004
    616.07'54—dc21
                                                                2003044710

Care has been taken to confirm the accuracy of the information presented and to describe generally accepted practices. However, the authors, editors, and publisher are not responsible for errors or omissions or for any consequences from application of the information in this book and make no warranty, express or implied, with respect to the content of the publication.

The authors, editors, and publisher have exerted every effort to ensure that drug selection and dosage set forth in this text are in accordance with the current recommendations and practice at the time of publication. However, in view of ongoing research, changes in government regulations, and the constant flow of information relating to drug therapy and drug reactions, the reader is urged to check the package insert for each drug for any change in indications and dosage and for added warnings and precautions. This is particularly important when the recommended agent is a new or infrequently employed drug.

Some drugs and medical devices presented in this publication have Food and Drug Administration (FDA) clearance for limited use in restricted research settings. It is the responsibility of the health care provider to ascertain the FDA status of each drug or device planned for use in his or her clinical practice.

LWW.com

Dedication

In memory of Barbara Bates, who pioneered a systemic, visual, and textual guide to physical examination and history taking used by students throughout the world.

Contents

Introduction

The *Pocket Guide to Physical Examination and History Taking,* 4/E is a concise, portable text that:

- Describes how to interview the patient and take the health history
- Provides an illustrated review of the physical examination
- Reminds students of common, typical findings
- Describes special techniques of assessment that students may need in specific instances
- Provides succinct aids to interpretation of selected findings

There are several ways to use the *Pocket Guide*:

- To review and remember the content of a health history.
- To review and rehearse the techniques of examination. This can be done while learning a single section and again while combining the approaches to several body systems or regions into an integrated examination (see Chap. 1).
- To review common variations of normal and selected abnormalities. Observations are keener and more precise when the examiner knows what to look, listen, and feel for.
- To look up special techniques as the need arises. Maneuvers such as doing an Allen test are included in the relevant sections of the examination and highlighted by a shaded blue bar.
- To look up additional information about possible findings, including abnormalities and standards of normal.

The *Pocket Guide* is not intended to serve as a primary text for learning the skills of taking a history or performing a physical examination. Its detail is insufficient for these purposes. It is intended instead as an aid for student review and recall and as a convenient, brief, and portable reference.

An Overview of Physical Examination and History Taking

Clinical Assessment: The Road Ahead

This chapter provides a road map to clinical proficiency in three critical areas: health history, physical examination, and the written record, or "write-up."

For adults, the comprehensive history includes *Identifying Data and Source of the History, Chief Complaint(s), Present Illness, Past History, Family History, Personal and Social History*, and *Review of Systems*. New patients in the office or hospital merit a *comprehensive health history;* however, in many situations a more flexible *focused*, or *problem-oriented*, *interview* is appropriate. The components of the comprehensive health history structure the patient's story and the format of your written record, but the order shown on pp. 2–3 should not dictate the sequence of the interview. Usually the interview will be more fluid and will follow the patient's leads and cues, as described in Chapter 2.

Distinguishing Subjective From Objective Data	
Subjective Data	**Objective Data**
What the patient tells you	What you detect during examination
The history, from Chief Complaint through Review of Systems	All physical examination findings

COMPONENTS OF THE HEALTH HISTORY

Identifying Data

- *Identifying data*—such as age, gender, occupation, marital status
- *Source of the history*—usually the patient, but can be family member, friend, letter of referral, or medical record
- If appropriate, establish *source of referral*, because a written report may be needed

Reliability

- Varies according to the patient's memory, trust, and mood

Chief Complaint(s)

- The one or more symptoms or concerns causing the patient to seek care

Present Illness

- Amplifies the *Chief Complaint*, describes how each symptom developed
- Includes patient's thoughts and feelings about the illness
- Pulls in relevant portions of the *Review of Systems* (see next page)
- May include *medications, allergies*, habits of *smoking and alcohol*, because these are frequently pertinent to the present illness

Past History

- Childhood illnesses
- Adult illnesses with dates for at least four categories: medical; surgical; obstetric/gynecologic; and psychiatric
- Includes health maintenance practices such as immunizations, screening tests, lifestyle issues, and home safety

Family History

- Outlines or diagrams age and health, or age and cause of death, of siblings, parents, and grandparents
- Documents presence or absence of specific illnesses in family, such as hypertension, coronary artery disease, etc.

(continued)

COMPONENTS OF THE HEALTH HISTORY (Continued)

Personal and Social History

■ Describes educational level, family of origin, current household, personal interests, and lifestyle

Review of Systems

■ Documents presence or absence of common symptoms related to each major body system

THE COMPREHENSIVE ADULT HEALTH HISTORY

As you elicit the adult health history, be sure to include the following data: date and time of history; identifying data, which include age, gender, marital status, and occupation; and reliability, which reflects the quality of information the patient provides.

Chief Complaint(s)

Quote the patient's own words. "My stomach hurts and I feel awful"; or "I have come for my regular checkup."

Present Illness

This section is a complete, clear, and chronologic account of the problems prompting the patient to seek care. It should include the problem's onset, the setting in which it has developed, its manifestations, and any treatments. Principal symptoms should be well characterized, with descriptions of (1) location; (2) quality; (3) quantity or severity; (4) timing, including onset, duration, and frequency; (5) setting in which they occur; (6) aggravating and relieving factors; and (7) associated manifestations.

In addition, list *medications,* including name, dose, route, and frequency of use; *allergies,* including *specific reactions* to each medication; *tobacco* use; and *alcohol* and *drug* use.

■ Past History

List *childhood illnesses,* then list *adult illnesses* in each of four areas:

- *Medical* (e.g., diabetes, hypertension, hepatitis, asthma, HIV), with dates of onset; also information about hospitalizations with dates

- *Surgical* (include dates, indications, and types of operations)

- *Obstetric/gynecologic* (provide obstetric history, menstrual history, birth control, sexual preference, any concerns about HIV infection)

- *Psychiatric* (include dates, diagnoses, hospitalizations, and treatments)

Also discuss *health maintenance,* including *immunizations,* such as tetanus, pertussis, diphtheria, polio, measles, rubella, mumps, influenza, hepatitis B, *Haemophilus influenza* type b, and pneumococcal vaccine; and *screening tests,* such as tuberculin tests, Pap smears, mammograms, stools for occult blood, and cholesterol tests, together with the results and the dates they were last performed.

■ Family History

Outline or diagram the age and health, or age and cause of death, of each immediate relative, including grandparents, parents, siblings, children, and grandchildren. Record if the following conditions are present or absent in the family: hypertension, coronary artery disease, elevated cholesterol levels, stroke, diabetes, thyroid or renal disease, cancer (specify type), arthritis, tuberculosis, asthma or lung disease, headache, seizure disorder, mental illness, suicide, alcohol or drug addiction, and allergies, as well as symptoms that the patient reports.

■ Personal and Social History

Include occupation and the last year of schooling; home situation and significant others; sources of stress, both recent and long-term; important life experiences, such as military service; leisure activities; religious affiliation and spiritual beliefs; and activities of daily living (ADLs). Also include lifestyle habits such as *exercise* and *diet, safety measures,* and *alternative health care* practices.

■ Review of Systems

These questions go from "head to toe." Start with a fairly general question. This allows you to shift to more specific questions about systems that may be of concern. For example, "How are your ears and hearing?" "How about your lungs and breathing?" "Any trouble with your heart?" "How is your digestion?" The *Review of Systems* questions may uncover problems that the patient overlooked. *Remember to move major health events to the Present Illness or Past History in your write-up.* Some clinicians do the *Review of Systems* during the physical examination. If the patient has only a few symptoms, this combination can be efficient. If he or she has multiple symptoms, the flow of both the history and the examination can be disrupted.

General. Usual weight, recent weight change, any clothes that fit more tightly or loosely than before; weakness, fatigue, fever.

Skin. Rashes, lumps, sores, itching, dryness, color change, changes in hair or nails.

Head, Eyes, Ears, Nose, Throat (HEENT). *Head:* Headache, head injury, dizziness, lightheadedness. *Eyes:* Vision, glasses or contact lenses, last examination, pain, redness, excessive tearing, double vision, blurred vision, spots, specks, flashing lights, glaucoma, cataracts. *Ears:* Hearing, tinnitus, vertigo, earache, infection, discharge. If hearing is decreased, use or nonuse of hearing aid. *Nose and* *sinuses:* Frequent colds, nasal stuffiness, discharge or itching, hay fever, nosebleeds, sinus trouble. ***Throat (or mouth and pharynx):*** Condition of teeth and gums; bleeding gums; dentures, if any, and how they fit; last dental examination; sore tongue; dry mouth; frequent sore throats; hoarseness.

Neck. Lumps, "swollen glands," goiter, pain, stiffness.

Breasts. Lumps, pain or discomfort, nipple discharge, self-examination practices.

Respiratory. Cough, sputum (color, quantity), hemoptysis, dyspnea, wheezing, pleurisy, last chest x-ray. You may wish to include asthma, bronchitis, emphysema, pneumonia, and tuberculosis.

Cardiovascular. Heart trouble, hypertension, rheumatic fever, heart murmurs, chest pain or discomfort, palpitations, dyspnea, orthopnea, paroxysmal nocturnal dyspnea, edema, past electrocardiographic or other heart test results.

Gastrointestinal. Trouble swallowing, heartburn, appetite, nausea, bowel movements, color and size of stools, change in bowel habits, rectal bleeding or black or tarry stools, hemorrhoids, constipation, diarrhea. Abdominal pain, food intolerance, excessive belching or passing of gas. Jaundice, liver or gallbladder trouble, hepatitis.

Urinary. Frequency of urination, polyuria, nocturia, urgency, burning or pain on urination, hematuria, urinary infections, kidney stones, incontinence; in males, reduced caliber or force of urinary stream, hesitancy, dribbling.

Genital. *Male:* Hernias, discharge from or sores on penis, testicular pain or masses, history of sexually transmitted diseases (STDs) and treatments, testicular self-examination practices. Sexual habits, interest, function, satisfaction, birth control methods, condom use, problems. Exposure to HIV infection. *Female:* Age at menarche; regularity, frequency, and duration of periods; amount of bleeding, bleeding between periods or after intercourse, last menstrual period; dysmenorrhea, premenstrual tension; age at menopause, menopausal symptoms, postmenopausal bleeding. In patients born before 1971, exposure to diethylstilbestrol (DES) from maternal use during pregnancy. Vaginal discharge, itching, sores, lumps, STDs and treatments. Number of pregnancies, number and type of deliveries, number of abortions (spontaneous and induced); complications of pregnancy; birth control methods. Sexual preference, interest, function, satisfaction, problems (including dyspareunia). Exposure to HIV infection.

Peripheral Vascular. Intermittent claudication, leg cramps, varicose veins, past clots in veins.

Musculoskeletal. Muscle or joint pains, stiffness, arthritis, gout, backache. If present, describe location of affected joints or muscles, any swelling, redness, pain, tenderness, stiffness, weakness, limitation of motion or activity; include timing of symptoms (e.g., morning or evening), duration, any history of trauma.

Neurologic. Fainting, blackouts, seizures, weakness, paralysis, numbness or loss of sensation, tingling or "pins and needles," tremors or other involuntary movements.

Hematologic. Anemia, easy bruising or bleeding, past transfusions and/or transfusion reactions.

Endocrine. Thyroid trouble, heat or cold intolerance, excessive sweating, excessive thirst or hunger, polyuria, change in glove or shoe size.

Psychiatric. Nervousness; tension; mood, including depression; memory change; suicide attempts, if relevant.

THE PHYSICAL EXAMINATION: APPROACH AND OVERVIEW

Conduct a *comprehensive physical examination* on most new patients or patients being admitted to the hospital. For more *problem-oriented*, or *focused, assessments*, the presenting complaints will dictate what segments you elect to perform.

The key to a thorough and accurate physical examination is developing a systematic sequence of examination. With a few months of practice, you will acquire your own routine sequence. Learn to be thorough without wasting time, systematic without being rigid, gentle yet not afraid to cause discomfort should it be required. In applying the techniques of inspection, palpation, auscultation, and percussion, the skillful clinician examines each body region, and at the same time senses the whole patient. *Minimize the number of times you ask the patient to change position* from supine to sitting, or standing to lying supine. For an overview of the physical examination, study the sequence that follows. *Note that clinicians vary as to where they place different segments, especially for the musculoskeletal and nervous systems.*

■ The Comprehensive Physical Examination

General Survey. Observe general state of health, height, build, and sexual development. Note posture, motor activity, and gait; dress, grooming, and personal hygiene; and any odors of the body or breath. Watch facial expressions and note manner, affect, and reactions to persons and things in the environment. Listen to the patient's manner of speaking and note the state of awareness or level of consciousness.

The survey continues throughout the history and examination.

Vital Signs. Measure height, weight, and blood pressure. Count pulse and respiratory rate. If indicated, measure body temperature.

The **patient is sitting** on the edge of the bed or examining table, unless this position is contraindicated. Stand in front of the patient, moving to either side as needed.

Skin. Observe the skin of the face and its characteristics. Identify any lesions, noting their location, distribution, arrangement, type, and color. Inspect and palpate the hair and nails. Study the patient's hands. Continue your assessment of the skin as you examine the other body regions.

HEENT. *Head:* Examine the hair, scalp, skull, and face. *Eyes:* Check visual acuity and screen the visual fields. Note position and alignment of the eyes. Observe the eyelids and inspect the sclera and conjunctiva of each eye. With oblique lighting, inspect each cornea, iris, and lens. Compare the pupils, and test their reactions to light. Assess extraocular movements. With an ophthalmoscope, inspect the ocular fundi. *Ears:* Inspect the auricles, canals, and drums. Check auditory acuity. If acuity is diminished, check lateralization (Weber test) and compare air and bone conduction (Rinne test). *Nose and sinuses:* Examine the external nose; using a

Darken the room to promote papillary dilation and visibility of the fundi.

light and nasal speculum, inspect nasal mucosa, septum, and turbinates. Palpate for tenderness of the frontal and maxillary sinuses. *Throat (or mouth and pharynx):* Inspect the lips, oral mucosa, gums, teeth, tongue, palate, tonsils, and pharynx. *(You may wish to assess the Cranial Nerves at this point in the examination.)*

Neck. Inspect and palpate the cervical lymph nodes. Note any masses or unusual pulsations in the neck. Feel for any deviation of the trachea. Observe sound and effort of the patient's breathing. Inspect and palpate the thyroid gland.

Move behind the sitting patient to feel the thyroid gland and to examine the back, posterior thorax, and lungs.

Back. Inspect and palpate the spine and muscles.

Posterior Thorax and Lungs. Inspect and palpate the spine and muscles of the *upper* back. Inspect, palpate, and percuss the chest. Identify the level of diaphragmatic dullness on each side. Listen to the breath sounds; identify any adventitious (or added) sounds, and, if indicated, listen to the transmitted voice sound (see p. 107).

Breasts, Axillae, and Epitrochlear Nodes. *Female:* Inspect the breasts with patient's arms relaxed, then elevated, and then with her hands pressed on her hips. *Male and Female:* Inspect the axillae and feel for the axillary nodes; feel for the epitrochlear nodes.

The patient is **still sitting.** Move to the front again.

A Note on the Musculoskeletal System: By now, you have made some preliminary observations of the musculoskeletal system. You have inspected the hands, surveyed the upper back, and, at least in women, made a fair estimate of the shoulders' range of motion (ROM). Use these and subsequent observations to decide whether a full musculoskeletal examination is warranted. If indicated, *with the patient still sitting,* examine the hands, arms, shoulders, neck, and temporomandibular joints. Inspect and palpate the joints and check their ROM. *(You may choose to examine upper extremity muscle bulk, tone, strength, and reflexes at this time, or you may decide to wait.)*

Palpate the breasts, while continuing your inspection.

○— **Anterior Thorax and Lungs.** Inspect, palpate, and percuss the chest. Listen to the breath sounds, any adventitious sounds, and, if indicated, transmitted voice sounds.

The patient position is supine. Ask the patient to lie down. Stand at the right side of the patient's bed.

○ **Cardiovascular System.** Observe the jugular venous pulsations, and measure the jugular venous pressure in relation to the sternal angle. Inspect and palpate the carotid pulsations. Listen for carotid bruits.

Elevate head of bed to about 30°, adjusting as necessary to see the jugular venous pulsations.

⊸ / ⊸ Inspect and palpate the precordium. Note the location, diameter, amplitude, and duration of the apical impulse. Listen at the apex and the lower sternal border with the bell of a stethoscope. Listen at each auscultatory area with the diaphragm. Listen for the first and second heart sounds and for physiologic splitting of the second heart sound. Listen for any abnormal heart sounds or murmurs.

Ask the patient to roll partly onto the left side while you listen at the apex. Then have the patient roll back to supine while you listen to the rest of the heart. The patient should sit, lean forward, and exhale while you listen for the murmur of aortic regurgitation.

⊸ **Abdomen.** Inspect, auscultate, and percuss. Palpate lightly, then deeply. Assess the liver and spleen by percussion and then palpation. Try to feel the kidneys and palpate the aorta and its pulsations. If you suspect kidney infection, percuss posteriorly over the costovertebral angles.

Lower the head of the bed to the flat position. **The patient should be supine.**

⊸ / ⊺ **Lower Extremities.** Examine the legs, assessing the systems (see next page) while the patient is still supine. Each of these three systems can be further assessed when the patient stands.

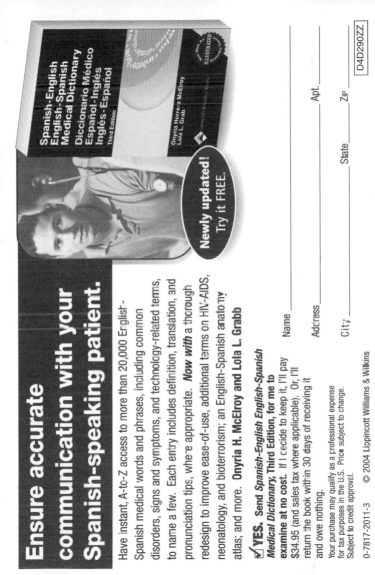

BUSINESS REPLY MAIL
FIRST-CLASS MAIL PERMIT NO. 31 HAGERSTOWN, MD

POSTAGE WILL BE PAID BY ADDRESSEE

LIPPINCOTT
WILLIAMS & WILKINS

DIRECT

PO BOX 1600
HAGERSTOWN MD 21741-9910

NO POSTAGE
NECESSARY
IF MAILED
IN THE
UNITED STATES

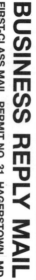

Examination	Patient Supine	Patient Standing
Peripheral Vascular System	Palpate femoral pulses, and, if indicated, popliteal pulses. Palpate inguinal lymph nodes. Inspect for lower extremity edema, discoloration, or ulcers. Palpate for pitting edema.	Inspect for varicose veins.
Musculoskeletal System	Note any deformities or enlarged joints. If indicated, palpate joints, check their ROM, and perform any necessary maneuvers.	Examine alignment of spine and its ROM, alignment of legs, and feet.
Genitalia and Hernias in Men		Examine penis and scrotal contents; check fro hernias.
Nervous System	Assess lower extremity muscle bulk, tone, and strength; also sensation and reflexes. Observe any abnormal movements.	Observe patient's gait and ability to walk heel-to-toe, walk on toes, walk on heels, hop in place, and do shallow knee bends. Do a Romberg test; check for pronator drift.

Nervous System. The complete examination of the nervous system also can be done at the end of the examination. It consists of five segments: *mental status, cranial nerves* (including funduscopic examination), *motor system, sensory system,* and *reflexes.*

The patient is **sitting or supine.**

Mental Status. If indicated and not done during the interview, assess orientation, mood, thought process, thought content, abnormal perceptions, insight and judgment, memory and attention, information and vocabulary, calculating abilities, abstract thinking, and constructional ability.

Cranial Nerves. If not already examined, check sense of smell, strength of the temporal and masseter muscles, corneal reflexes, facial movements, gag reflex, and strength of the trapezia and sternomastoidal muscles.

Motor System. Muscle bulk, tone, and strength of major muscle groups. *Cerebellar function:* rapid alternating movements (RAMs), point-to-point movements, such as finger-to-nose (F→N) and heel-to-shin (H→S); gait.

Sensory System. Pain, temperature, light touch, vibrations, and discrimination. Compare right with left sides and distal with proximal areas on the limbs.

Reflexes. Include biceps, triceps, brachioradialis, patellar, Achilles deep tendon reflexes; also plantar reflexes or Babinski reflex (see p. 288).

Additional Examinations. The *rectal* and *genital* examinations are often performed at the end of the physical examination. Patient positioning is as indicated.

Rectal Examination in Men. Inspect the sacrococcygeal and perianal areas. Palpate the anal canal, rectum, and prostate. If the patient cannot stand, examine the genitalia before doing the rectal examination.

The patient is **lying on his left side** for the rectal examination.

Genital and Rectal Examination in Women. Examine the external genitalia, vagina, and cervix. Obtain a Pap smear. Palpate the uterus and adnexa. Do a rectovaginal and rectal examination.

The patient is **supine in the lithotomy position.** Sit during the examination with the speculum, then stand during bimanual examination of uterus, adnexa, and rectum.

RECORDING YOUR FINDINGS

Your written record organizes the information from the history and physical examination and should clearly communicate the patient's clinical issues to all members of the health care team. Your record also should facilitate clinical reasoning and convey essential information to other consultants and providers.

TIPS FOR A CLEAR AND ACCURATE WRITE-UP

- Write the record as soon as possible, before the data fade from your memory. At first, you may want to take notes when talking with the patient. As you gain experience, however, work toward recording the *Present Illness,* the *Past Medical History,* the *Family History,* the *Personal and Social History,* and the *Review of Systems* in final form during the interview. Leave spaces to fill in details later.
- During the *physical examination,* make note immediately of specific measurements such as blood pressure and heart rate. Because recording multiple items does tend to interrupt the flow of the examination, you will soon learn to remember your findings and record them after you have finished.

Order of the Write-up

- Pay special attention to the *order* and *degree of detail.* Remember that if handwritten, a good record is always legible!
- Make the order consistent and obvious so that finding specific information is easy. Keep subjective data in the history, and do not let them stray into the physical examination.
- Offset your headings and use indentations and spacing to make your organization clear. Use asterisks and underlines to emphasize important points.
- Arrange the *Present Illness* chronologically, starting with the current episode and then filling in relevant background information. For example, if a patient with long-standing diabetes is hospitalized in a coma, begin with the events leading up to the coma and then summarize the past history of the patient's diabetes.

Degree of Detail

- The *degree of detail* should be pertinent to the subject or problem but not redundant.

THE PHYSICAL EXAMINATION: SUMMARY OF SUGGESTED SEQUENCE

- General survey
- Vital signs
- Skin: upper torso, anterior and posterior
- Head and neck, including thyroid and lymph nodes
- *Optional:* Nervous system (mental status, cranial nerves, upper extremity motor strength, bulk, tone; cerebellar function)
- Thorax and lungs
- Breasts
- Musculoskeletal as indicated: upper extremities
- Cardiovascular, including JVP, carotid upstrokes and bruits, PMI, etc.
- Cardiovascular, for S_3 and murmur of mitral stenosis
- Nervous system: lower extremity
- Musculoskeletal, as indicated
- *Optional:* Skin, anterior and posterior
- *Optional:* Nervous system, including gait
- *Optional:* Musculoskeletal, comprehensive
- *Women:* Pelvic and rectal examination
- *Men:* Prostate and rectal examination
- Cardiovascular, for murmur of aortic insufficiency
- *Optional:* Thorax and lungs — anterior
- Breasts and axillae
- Abdomen
- Peripheral vascular; *Optional:* Skin-lower torso and extremities

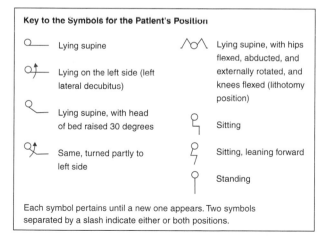

Key to the Symbols for the Patient's Position

Lying supine

Lying on the left side (left lateral decubitus)

Lying supine, with head of bed raised 30 degrees

Same, turned partly to left side

Lying supine, with hips flexed, abducted, and externally rotated, and knees flexed (lithotomy position)

Sitting

Sitting, leaning forward

Standing

Each symbol pertains until a new one appears. Two symbols separated by a slash indicate either or both positions.

Interviewing and the Health History

The health history interview is a conversation with a purpose. Unlike social conversation, in which you express your own needs and interests with responsibility only for yourself, the primary goal of the clinician–patient interview is to improve the well-being of the patient. The purpose of conversation with a patient is threefold: to establish a trusting and supportive relationship, to gather information, and to offer information.

The interviewing process differs significantly from the format for the health history presented in Chapter 1. Both are fundamental to your work with patients, but each serves a different purpose. The health history format is a structured framework for organizing patient information in written or verbal form.

The interviewing process that actually generates these pieces of information is more fluid. It requires knowledge of the information you need to obtain, the ability to elicit accurate and detailed information, and interpersonal skills that allow you to respond to the patient's feelings.

For new patients, you will do a *comprehensive health history*, described for adults in Chapter 1. For other patients who seek care for a specific complaint, such as painful urination, a more limited interview, tailored to that specific problem may be indicated, sometimes called a *problem-oriented history*.

■ Getting Ready: The Approach to the Interview

Interviewing patients to obtain a health history requires planning.

- **Take time for self-reflection.** As clinicians, we encounter a wide variety of people, each of whom is unique. Because we bring our own values, assumptions, and biases to every encounter, we must look inward to clarify how our expectations and reactions affect what we hear and how we behave. *Self-reflection brings a deepening personal awareness to our work with patients and is one of the most rewarding aspects of providing patient care.*

- **Review the chart.** Before seeing the patient, review his or her medical record, or chart. It often provides valuable information about past diagnoses and treatments; however, data may be incomplete or even disagree with what you learn from the patient. Do not let the chart prevent you from developing new approaches or ideas.

- **Set goals for the interview.** Clarify your goals for the interview. A clinician must balance provider-centered goals with patient-centered goals. The clinician's task is to consider these multiple agendas.

- **Review clinician behavior and appearance.** Consciously or not, you send messages through both your words and your behavior. Posture, gestures, eye contact, and tone of voice all can express interest, attention, acceptance, and understanding. The skilled interviewer seems calm and unhurried, even when time is limited. Reactions that betray disapproval, embarrassment, impatience, or boredom block communication. Patients find cleanliness, neatness, conservative dress, and a nametag reassuring.

- **Improve the environment.** Make the setting as private and comfortable as possible. Always consider the patient's privacy. Pull shut any bedside curtains. Suggest moving to an empty room rather than having a conversation that can be overheard.

- **Take notes.** Jot down short phrases, specific dates, or words rather than trying to put them into a final format. Maintain good eye contact, and whenever the patient is talking about sensitive or disturbing material, put down your pen.

■ Learning About the Patient: The Process of Interviewing

In general, an interview moves through several stages. *Throughout this sequence, you, as the clinician, must always stay attuned to the patient's feelings, help the patient express them, respond to their content, and validate their significance.*

Whether the interview is comprehensive or focused, be sure to focus on the patient's feelings and affect.

Greet the patient and establish rapport. As you begin, *greet the patient* by name and introduce yourself, giving your name. If possible, shake hands. If this is the first contact, explain your role, including your status as a student and how you will be involved in the patient's care. Using a title to address the patient (e.g., Mr. O'Neil, Ms. Wu) is always best. Avoid first names unless you have specific permission from the patient.

Whenever visitors are present, it is important to *maintain confidentiality.* Let the patient decide if visitors or family members should remain in the room, and ask for the patient's permission before conducting the interview in front of them.

Attend to the patient's comfort. Ask how he or she is feeling and if you are coming at a convenient time. Look for signs of discomfort, such as frequent changes of position or facial expressions that show pain or anxiety. Arranging the bed may make the patient more comfortable.

Consider the best way to *arrange the room.* Choose a distance that facilitates conversation and good eye contact. Try to sit at eye level with the patient. Move any physical barriers between you and the patient, such as desks or bedside tables, out of the way.

Give the patient your undivided attention. Try not to look down to take notes or read the chart, and spend enough time on small talk to put the patient at ease.

Invite the patient's story. Begin with **open-ended questions** that allow full freedom of response. "What concerns bring you here today?" or "How can I help you?" These questions do not restrict the patient to a limited and minimally informative "yes" or "no" answer. *Listen to the patient's answers without interrupting.*

Some patients may not have a specific complaint or problem. *It is still important to start with the patient's story.* Helpful open-ended questions are "Do you have any special concerns for our appointment today?" and "What brings you in for health care now?"

Train yourself to *follow the patient's leads.* Good interviewing techniques include using verbal and nonverbal cues that prompt patients to recount their stories spontaneously. Use *continuers,* especially at the outset, such as nodding your head and using phrases such as "Uh huh," "Go on," and "I see."

Establish the agenda for the interview. It is important to identify both your own and the patient's issues at the beginning of the encounter. Often, you may need to focus the interview by asking the patient which problem is most pressing. For example, "Which problem are you most concerned about today?"

Expand and clarify the health history (the patient's perspective). Each symptom has attributes that must be clarified, including context, associations, and chronology, especially for pain. For all symptoms, it is critical to understand fully their essential characteristics. *Always elicit the seven features of every symptom.*

Be sure to *use language that is understandable and appropriate* to the patient. Technical language confuses the patient and often blocks communication. Whenever possible, *use the patient's words, making sure you clarify their meaning.*

THE SEVEN ATTRIBUTES OF A SYMPTOM

1. **Location.** Where is it? Does it radiate?
2. **Quality.** What is it like?
3. **Quantity or severity.** How bad is it? (For pain, ask for a rating on a scale of 1–10.)
4. **Timing.** When did (does) it start? How long did (does) it last? How often did (does) it come?
5. **Setting in which it occurs.** Include environmental factors, personal activities, emotional reactions, or other circumstances that may have contributed to the illness.
6. **Remitting or exacerbating factors.** Does anything make it better or worse?
7. **Associated manifestations.** Have you noticed anything else that accompanies it?

Learn to facilitate the patient's story by using different types of questions and the techniques of skilled interviewing described on pp. 23–26. Often you will need to *use directed questions* (see p. 24) that ask for specific information the patient has not already offered. *In general, the patient interview moves back and forth from an open-ended question to a directed question and then on to another open-ended question.*

Establishing the sequence and time course of the patient's symptoms is important. You can encourage a chronologic account by asking such questions as "What then?" or "What happened next?"

Generate and test diagnostic hypotheses (the clinician's perspective). As you listen to the patient's concerns, you will begin to *generate and test diagnostic hypotheses* about what disease process might be the cause. Identifying the various attributes of the patient's symptoms and pursuing specific details are fundamental to recognizing patterns of disease and differentiating one disease from another.

Create a shared understanding of the problem. The *disease/illness model* helps you understand the difference between your perspective and the patient's perspective. In this model, *disease* is the explanation that the *clinician* brings to the symptoms. It is the way that the clinician organizes what he or she learns from the patient into a coherent picture that leads to a clinical diagnosis and treatment plan. *Illness* can be defined as how the *patient* experiences symptoms. *The health history interview needs to take into account both of these views of reality.*

Learning how patients perceive illness means asking patient-centered questions in the six domains listed below. This is crucial to patient satisfaction, effective health care, and patient follow-through.

EXPLORING THE PATIENT'S PERSPECTIVE

- The patient's thoughts about the nature and the cause of the problem
- The patient's feelings, especially fears, about the problem
- The patient's expectations of the clinician and health care
- The effect of the problem on the patient's life
- Prior personal or family experiences that are similar
- Therapeutic responses the patient has already tried

Negotiate a plan. Learning about the disease and conceptualizing the illness give you and the patient the basis for planning further evaluation (physical examination, laboratory tests, consultations, etc.).

Plan for follow-up and closing. Make sure the patient understands the agreed-upon plans you have developed. You can say, "We need to stop now. Do you have any questions about what we've covered?" Review future evaluation, treatments, and follow-up. Give the patient a chance to ask any final questions.

■ Facilitating the Patient's Story: The Techniques of Skilled Interviewing

Skilled interviewing requires the use of specific learnable techniques. Practice these techniques and find ways to be observed or recorded so that you can receive feedback on your progress.

Active Listening. This requires listening closely to what the patient is communicating, being aware of the patient's emotional state, and using verbal and nonverbal skills to encourage the speaker to continue and expand.

Adaptive Questioning. Learn to adapt your questioning to the patient's verbal and nonverbal cues.

ADAPTIVE QUESTIONING: OPTIONS FOR CLARIFYING THE PATIENT'S STORY

- Directed questioning—from general to specific
- Questioning to elicit a graded response
- Asking a series of questions, one at a time
- Offering multiple choices for answers
- Clarifying what the patient means

Directed questioning draws the patient's attention to specific areas of the history. *Proceed from the general to the specific. Directed questions should not be leading questions* that call for a "yes" or "no" answer: not "Did your stools look like tar?" but "Please describe your stools."

Ask questions that require *a graded response* rather than a single answer. "What physical activity do you do that makes you short of breath?" is better than "Do you get short of breath climbing stairs?" Be sure to *ask one question at a time.* Try "Do you have any of the following problems?" Be sure to pause and establish eye contact as you list each problem.

Sometimes patients seem unable to describe symptoms. *Offer multiple-choice answers.*

For patients using words that are ambiguous, *request clarification,* as in "Tell me exactly what you meant by 'the flu.' "

Nonverbal Communication. Being sensitive to nonverbal messages allows you both to "read the patient" more effectively and to send messages of your own. Pay close attention to eye contact, facial expression, posture, head position and movement such as shaking or nodding, interpersonal distance, and placement of the arms or legs, such as crossed, neutral, or open. Physical contact (like placing your hand on the patient's arm) can convey empathy or help the patient gain control of feelings. You also can mirror the patient's *paralanguage,* or qualities of speech such as pacing, tone, and volume, to increase rapport.

Facilitation. Posture, actions, or words encourage the patient to say more but do not specify the topic. Nod your head or remain silent. Lean forward, make eye contact, and use continuers like "Mm-hmm," "Go on," or "I'm listening."

Echoing. Repetition of the patient's words encourages the patient to express both factual details and feelings.

Empathic Responses. Patients may express—with or without words—feelings they have not consciously acknowledged. *To empathize with your patient you must first identify his or her feelings.* Inquire about them rather than assuming how the patient feels.

Respond with understanding and acceptance. Responses may be as simple as "I understand," "That sounds upsetting," or "You seem sad." Empathy also may be nonverbal—for example, offering a tissue to a crying patient.

Validation. An important way to make a patient feel accepted is to legitimize or validate his or her emotional experience.

Reassurance. You may fall into reassuring the patient about the wrong thing. Premature reassurance may block further disclosures, especially if the patient feels that exposing anxiety is a weakness. *The first step to effective reassurance is identifying and accepting the patient's feelings without offering reassurance at that moment.*

Summarization. Giving a capsule summary lets the patient know that you have been listening carefully. It also can identify what you know and what you don't know. Summarization also allows you to organize your clinical reasoning and to convey your thinking to the patient, which makes the relationship more collaborative.

Highlighting Transitions. Tell patients when you are changing directions during the interview. This gives patients a greater sense of control.

■ Adapting Interviewing Techniques to Specific Situations

Always remember the importance of listening to the patient and clarifying the patient's agenda.

Silent Patient. Silence has many meanings and purposes. Watch closely for nonverbal cues (e.g., difficulty controlling emotions). You may need to shift your inquiry to symptoms of depression or begin an exploratory mental status examination. Silence may be the patient's response to how you are asking questions. Are you asking too many direct questions? Have you offended the patient?

Talkative Patient. With a garrulous, rambling patient, several techniques are helpful. For the first 5 or 10 minutes, listen closely. Does the patient seem obsessively detailed or unduly anxious? Is there a flight of ideas or disorganized thought process? Try to focus on what seems most important to the patient. "You've described many concerns. Let's focus on the hip pain first. Can you tell me what it feels like?"

Anxious Patient. Watch for nonverbal and verbal cues. Anxious patients may sit tensely, fidgeting. They may sigh frequently. Reflect your impression to the patient and encourage him or her to discuss any underlying concerns.

Crying Patient. Usually crying is therapeutic, as is quiet acceptance of the patient's distress. Make a facilitating or supportive remark like "I'm glad that you got that out."

Confusing Patient. Some patients have *multiple symptoms* or a somatization disorder. Focus on the meaning or function of the symptom and guide the interview into a psychosocial assessment. At other times you may be baffled, frustrated, and confused. The history is vague and difficult to understand, and patients may describe symptoms in bizarre terms. Try to learn more about the unusual symptoms. Watch for delirium in acutely ill or intoxicated patients and for dementia in the elderly. When you suspect a psychiatric or neurologic disorder, shift to a mental status examination, focusing on level of consciousness, orientation, and memory.

Angry or Disruptive Patient. Many patients have reasons to be angry: they are ill, they have suffered a loss, they lack accustomed control over their own lives, and they feel relatively powerless. They may direct this anger toward you. Accept angry feelings from patients and allow them to express such emotions without getting angry in return. Validate their feelings without agreeing with their reasons. "I understand that you felt very frustrated by the long wait and answering the same questions over and over." Some angry patients become hostile and disruptive. Before approaching them, alert security. It is especially important to stay calm, appear accepting, and avoid being challenging. Keep your posture relaxed and nonthreatening. Once you have established rapport, gently suggest moving to a different location.

Patient With a Language Barrier. The ideal interpreter is a neutral objective person familiar with both languages and cultures. Avoid using family members or friends as interpreters: confidentiality may be violated. As you begin working with the interpreter, *make questions clear, short, and simple.* Speak directly to the patient. Bilingual written questionnaires are invaluable.

Patient With Personal Problems. Patients may ask you for advice about personal problems outside the range of health. Letting the patient talk through the problem with you is usually much more valuable and therapeutic than any answer you could give. The following box offers ways to adapt the interview to particular types of patients.

GUIDELINES FOR WORKING
WITH AN INTERPRETER

- Choose a professional interpreter in preference to a hospital worker, volunteer, or family member. Use the interpreter as a resource for cultural information.
- Orient the interpreter to the components you plan to cover in the interview; include reminders to translate everything the patient says.
- Arrange the room so that you and the patient have eye contact and can read each other's nonverbal cues.
- Seat the interpreter next to you and allow the interpreter and the patient to establish rapport.
- Address the patient directly. Reinforce your questions with nonverbal behaviors.
- Keep sentences short and simple. Focus on the most important concepts to communicate.
- Verify mutual understanding by asking the patient to report back what he or she has heard.
- Be patient. The interview will take more time and may provide less information.

Patient With Reading Problems. Assess ability to read. Some patients may try to hide their reading problems. Ask the patient to read whatever instructions you have written. Simply handing the patient written material upside-down to see if the patient turns it around may settle the question.

Patient With Impaired Hearing. Find out the patient's preferred method of communicating. Patients may use American Sign Language, a unique language with its own syntax, or various other communication forms combining signs and speech. Determine whether the patient identifies with the Deaf or Hearing culture. Handwritten questions and answers may be the best solution. When patients have *partial hearing impairment* or can *read lips*, face them directly, in good light. If the patient has a *unilateral hearing loss*, sit on the hearing side. If the patient has a *hearing aid*, make sure it is working. Eliminate background noise such as television.

Patient With Impaired Vision. Shake hands to establish contact and explain who you are and why you are there.

If the room is unfamiliar, orient the patient to the surroundings.

Patient With Limited Intelligence. Patients of moderately limited intelligence usually can give adequate histories. Pay special attention to the patient's schooling and ability to function independently. How far has the patient gone in school? If he or she didn't finish, why not? The sexual history is equally important and often overlooked. Assess simple calculations, vocabulary, memory, and abstract thinking. For patients with severe mental retardation, obtain the history from the family or caregivers. Avoid "talking down" or using condescending behavior.

Poor Historian. Some patients cannot give their own histories. Try to find a third person who can tell the story. You may discover surprising and important information. For patients who are mentally competent, you must obtain their consent before you talk about their health with others.

■ Special Aspects of Interviewing

Cultural Competence. As you provide care for an ever-expanding and diverse group of patients, it is important to understand how culture shapes not just the patient's beliefs, but your own. *Culture* is a system of shared ideas, rules, and meanings that influences how we view the world, experience it emotionally, and behave in relation to other people. This definition of culture is broader than the term *ethnicity*. The influence of culture is not limited to minority groups—it is relevant to everyone.

Self-awareness. As clinicians, we face the task of bringing our own values and biases to a conscious level. *Values* are the standards we use to measure our own and others' beliefs and behaviors. *Biases* are the attitudes or feelings that we attach to perceived differences; for example, the way an individual relates to time, which can be a culturally determined phenomenon. Are you always on time—a positive value in the dominant Western culture? Or do you tend to run a little late? How do you feel about people whose habits are opposite to yours? Think about the role of physical appearance. Do you consider yourself thin, midsize, or heavy? How do you feel about people who have different weights?

Enhanced Communication and Learning From the Patient. Maintain an open, respectful, and inquiring attitude. "What did you hope to get from this visit?" If you have established rapport and trust, patients will be willing to teach you. Be ready to acknowledge your ignorance or bias. "I mistakenly made assumptions about you that are not right. I apologize. Would you be willing to tell me more about yourself and your future goals?"

Do some reading. Go to movies that are made in different countries. Learn about different consumer health agendas.

Collaborative Partnerships. Communication based on trust, respect, and a willingness to reexamine assumptions helps allow patients to express concerns that may run counter to the dominant culture. You, the clinician, must be willing to listen to and to validate these feelings, and not let your own feelings prevent you from exploring painful areas. You also must be willing to reexamine your beliefs.

The Alcohol and Drug History. Clinicians should routinely ask about current and past use of alcohol or drugs, patterns of use, and family history. "What do you like to drink?" or "Tell me about your use of alcohol" are good opening questions that avoid the easy yes or no response. The most widely used screening questions are the CAGE questions about **C**utting down, **A**nnoyance if criticized, **G**uilty feelings, and **E**ye-openers.

Two or more affirmative answers to the CAGE Questionnaire suggest alcoholism. Ask more questions about blackouts (loss of memory for events during drinking), seizures, accidents or injuries while drinking, job loss, marital conflict, or legal problems. Also ask specifically about drinking while driving or operating machinery.

THE CAGE QUESTIONNAIRE

- Have you ever felt the need to **Cut down** on drinking?
- Have you ever felt **Annoyed** by criticism of drinking?
- Have you ever felt **Guilty** about drinking?
- Have you ever taken a drink first thing in the morning (**Eye-opener**) to steady your nerves or get rid of a hangover?

(Adapted from Mayfield D, McLeod G, Hall P: The CAGE questionnaire: Validation of a new alcoholism screening instrument. Am J Psychiatry 131: 1121–1123, 1974.)

Questions about drugs are similar. "How much marijuana do you use? Cocaine? Heroin? Amphetamines?" (ask about each one by name). "How about prescription drugs such as sleeping pills?" "Diet pills?" "Painkillers?" With adolescents, it may be helpful to ask about substance use by friends or family members first. "A lot of young people are using drugs these days. How about at your school? Your friends?"

The Sexual History. You can introduce questions about sexual function and practices at multiple points in a patient's history. An orienting sentence or two is often helpful. "Now I'd like to ask you some questions about your sexual health and practices" or "I routinely ask all patients about their sexual function."

- "When was the last time you had intimate physical contact with anyone?" "Did that contact include sexual intercourse?"

- "Do you have sex with men, women, or both?" The health implications of heterosexual, homosexual, or bisexual experiences are significant.

- "How many sexual partners have you had in the last 6 months?" "In the last 5 years?" "In your lifetime?"

- Because no explicit risk factors may be present, it is important to ask all patients "Do you have any concerns about HIV disease or AIDS?" Ask also about routine use of condoms.

Domestic and Physical Violence. Many authorities recommend the routine screening of all female patients for domestic violence. Start this part of the interview with general "normalizing" questions: "Because abuse is common in many women's lives, I've begun to ask about it routinely." "Are there times in your relationships that you feel unsafe or afraid?"

Consider physical abuse in the following settings:

- If injuries are unexplained, seem inconsistent with the patient's story, are concealed by the patient, or cause embarrassment

- If the patient has delayed getting treatment for trauma

- If there is a past history of repeated injuries or "accidents"

- If the patient or a person close to the patient has a history of alcohol or drug abuse

Also be suspicious if a partner tries to dominate the interview, will not leave the room, or seems unusually anxious or solicitous.

Death and the Dying Patient. You will need to work through your own feelings with the help of reading and discussion. Kubler-Ross has described five stages in a person's response to loss or the anticipatory grief of impending death: denial and isolation, anger, bargaining, depression or sadness, and acceptance. These stages may occur sequentially or overlap in different combinations.

Dying patients rarely want to talk about their illnesses all the time, nor do they wish to confide in everyone they meet. Give them opportunities to talk and then listen receptively, but if they prefer to stay at a social level, you need not feel like a failure.

Understanding the patient's wishes about treatment at the end of life is an important part of a clinician's role. Even if discussions of death and dying are difficult for you, you must learn to ask specific questions. Ask about "*DNR status*" (Do

Not Resuscitate). Find out about the patient's frame of reference. "What experiences have you had with the death of a close friend or relative?" "What do you know about cardiopulmonary resuscitation (CPR)?" Assure them that relieving pain and taking care of their other spiritual and physical needs will be a priority.

Encourage any adult, but especially the elderly or chronically ill, to establish a *health care proxy,* an individual who can act for the patient in life-threatening situations.

Sexuality in the Clinician–Patient Relationship. The emotional and physical intimacy of the clinician–patient relationship may lead to sexual feelings. If you become aware of such feelings, accept them as a normal human response, and bring them to the conscious level so they will not affect your behavior. Denying these feelings makes it more likely for you to act inappropriately. *Any* sexual contact or romantic relationship with patients is *unethical;* keep your relationship with the patient within professional bounds and seek help if you need it.

■ Ethical Considerations

Fundamental maxims are as follows:

- *Nonmaleficence* or *primum non nocere,* commonly stated as "First, do no harm"

- *Beneficence,* or the dictum that the clinician needs to "do good" for the patient. As clinicians, our actions need to be motivated by what is in the patient's best interest.

- *Autonomy,* or that patients have the right to determine what is in their own best interest

- *Confidentiality,* meaning that we are obligated not to tell others what we learn from our patients

The Tavistock Principles guide behavior in health care for both individuals and institutions.

THE TAVISTOCK PRINCIPLES

Rights: People have a right to health and health care.

Balance: Care of individual patients is central, but the health of populations is also our concern.

Comprehensiveness: In addition to treating illness, we have an obligation to ease suffering, minimize disability, prevent disease, and promote health.

Cooperation: Health care succeeds only if we cooperate with those we serve, each other, and those in other sectors.

Improvement: Improving health care is a serious and continuing responsibility.

Safety: Do no harm.

Openness: Being open, honest, and trustworthy is vital in health care.

Interviewing Aging Patients

Learn how the elderly and those with chronic illness function in terms of daily activities, namely: physical activities of daily living (ADLs) and instrumental activities of daily living (IADLs).

ACTIVITIES OF DAILY LIVING (ADLs)

Physical ADLs	Instrumental ADLs
Bathing	Using the telephone
Dressing	Shopping
Toileting	Preparing food
Transfers	Housekeeping
Continence	Laundry
Feeding	Transportation
	Taking medicine
	Managing money

Beginning the Physical Examination: General Survey and Vital Signs

Survey the patient's general appearance and measure height and weight. Learn to measure the *Body Mass Index (BMI)*, which incorporates estimated but more accurate measurements of body fat than weight alone. More than 50% of U.S. adults are overweight (BMI >25); nearly 25% are obese (BMI >30). These excesses are proven risk factors for diabetes, heart disease, stroke, hypertension, osteoarthritis, and some forms of cancer.

Calculating BMI. Measure the *waist circumference* just above the hip bones. The patient may have excess body fat if the waist measures ≥35 inches for women or ≥40 inches for men.

If the BMI falls *above 25*, engage the patient in a 24-hour dietary recall and compare the intake of food groups and number of servings per day with current recommendations. Or choose a screening tool and provide appropriate counseling or referral. If the BMI falls *below 17*, be concerned about possible anorexia nervosa, bulimia, or other medical conditions (see Tables 3-1 and 3-2, pp. 50–51).

To measure BMI, choose the method most suited to your practice.

Methods to Calculate Body Mass Index (BMI)

Unit of Measure	Method of Calculation
Weight *in pounds,* height *in inches*	(1) Body Mass Index Chart (see p. 50) (2) Body Mass Index Nomogram (see p. 51) (3) $\dfrac{\left(\dfrac{\text{Weight (lbs)} \times 700^\star}{\text{Height (inches)}}\right)}{\text{Height (inches)}}$
Weight *in kilograms,* height *in meters squared*	(4) $\dfrac{\text{Weight (kg)}}{\text{Height (m}^2)}$
Either	(5) "BMI Calculator" at website www.nhlbisupport.com/bmi

*Several organizations use 704.5, but the variation in BMI is negligible.

Conversion formulas: 2.2 lbs = 1 kg; 1.0 inch = 2.54 cm; 100 cm = 1 meter

(Source: National Institute of Diabetes and Digestive and Kidney Diseases. www.niddk.nih.gov/health/nutrit/pubs/statobes.htm, Accessed 2/1/01.)

THE HEALTH HISTORY

Common or Concerning Symptoms

■ Changes in weight
■ Fatigue and weakness
■ Fever and chills

Changes in Weight. *Weight gain* occurs when caloric intake exceeds caloric expenditure over time. It also may reflect abnormal accumulation of body fluids. Good opening questions include "How often do you check your weight?" "How is it compared to a year ago?"

Weight loss has many causes: decreased food intake, dysphagia, vomiting, and insufficient supplies of food;

defective absorption of nutrients; increased metabolic requirements; and loss of nutrients through the urine, feces, or injured skin. Be alert for signs of malnutrition.

Fatigue and Weakness. *Fatigue* is a relatively nonspecific symptom with many causes. Use open-ended questions to explore the attributes of the patient's fatigue, and encourage the patient to fully describe what he or she is experiencing.

Weakness differs from fatigue. It denotes a demonstrable loss of muscle power and will be discussed later with other neurologic symptoms.

Fever and Chills. Ask about fever if patients have an acute or chronic illness. Find out whether the patient has used a thermometer to measure the temperature. Distinguish between subjective *chilliness* and a *shaking chill,* with shivering throughout the body and chattering of teeth.

Focus your questions on the timing of the illness and its associated symptoms. Become familiar with patterns of infectious diseases that may affect your patient. Inquire about travel, contact with sick people, or other unusual exposures. Be sure to inquire about medications, since they may cause fever. In contrast, recent ingestion of aspirin, acetaminophen, corticosteroids, and nonsteroidal anti-inflammatory drugs may mask it.

HEALTH PROMOTION AND COUNSELING

Important Topics for Health Promotion and Counseling

- Optimal weight and nutrition
- Exercise
- Blood pressure and diet

Optimal Weight and Nutrition. Less than half of U.S. adults maintain a healthy weight (BMI ≥19 but ≤25). Obesity has increased in every segment of the population. More than 50% of people with type 2 diabetes and roughly 20% of those with hypertension or elevated cholesterol levels are overweight or obese. Increasing obesity in children has been linked to rising rates of childhood diabetes.

Explain the components of a healthy diet and encourage appropriately sized servings from each of the five major food groups: grains such as bread, cereal, rice, and pasta; fruits; vegetables; dairy products; and meat and beans. See "Aids to Interpretation" for specific suggestions.

Exercise. Thirty minutes of moderate activity, defined as walking 2 miles in 30 minutes on most days of the week or its equivalent, is recommended. Patients can increase exercise by such simple measures as parking further away from their place of work or using stairs instead of elevators.

Blood Pressure and Diet. Regular and frequent exercise, decreased sodium and increased potassium intake, and maintenance of a healthy weight will reduce the risk of developing hypertension as well as lower blood pressure in adults who are already hypertensive.

TECHNIQUES OF EXAMINATION

■ Beginning the Examination: Setting the Stage

Preparing for the Physical Examination

- Reflect on your approach to the patient.
- Decide on the scope of the examination.
- Choose the examination sequence.
- Adjust the lighting and the environment.
- Make the patient comfortable.

Think through your approach, your professional demeanor, and how to make the patient comfortable and relaxed. *Wash your hands in the patient's presence before beginning.*

Approaching the Patient. Let the patient know you are a student, and try to appear calm, organized, and competent, even if you feel differently. If you forget to do part of the examination, this is not uncommon, especially at first! Simply examine those areas out of sequence but smoothly.

Scope of the Examination: *How Complete Should It Be?* Choose whether to do a *comprehensive* or *focused* examination.

■ A *comprehensive physical examination* is a source of fundamental and personalized knowledge about the patient and strengthens the clinician–patient relationship.

■ For the *focused examination,* select the methods relevant to assessing the problem as precisely and carefully as possible.

Choosing the Examination Sequence, Examining Position, and Handedness. The sequence of the comprehensive or focused examination should maximize the patient's comfort, avoid unnecessary changes in position, and enhance the clinician's efficiency. In general, move from "head to toe." An important goal as a student is to develop your own sequence with these principles in mind. See Chapter 1 for a suggested examination sequence.

This book recommends examining the patient from the patient's right side. It is more reliable to estimate jugular venous pressure from the right, the palpating hand rests more comfortably on the apical impulse, the right kidney is more frequently palpable than the left, and examining tables are frequently positioned to accommodate a right-handed approach. To examine the *supine patient,* you can examine the head, neck, and anterior chest. Then roll the patient onto each side to listen to the lungs, examine the back, and inspect the skin. Roll the patient back and finish the rest of the examination with the patient again supine.

Adjusting Lighting and the Environment. Adjust the bed to a convenient height (be sure to lower it when finished!). Ask the patient to move toward you if this makes it easier.

Good lighting and a quiet environment are important. *Tangential lighting* is optimal for structures such as the jugular venous pulse, the thyroid gland, and the apical impulse of the heart. It throws contours, elevations, and depressions, whether moving or stationary, into sharper relief.

Promoting the Patient's Comfort. Show concern for privacy and modesty.

■ Close nearby doors and draw curtains before beginning.

■ Acquire the art of *draping the patient* with the gown or draw sheet as you learn each examination segment in future chapters. *The goal is to visualize one body area at a time.*

■ As you proceed, keep the patient informed, as when checking for the femoral pulse. Also try to gauge how much the patient wants to know.

■ Make sure your instructions to the patient at each step are courteous and clear.

■ Watch the patient's facial expression and even ask "Is it okay?" as you move through the examination.

When you have finished, tell the patient your general impressions and what to expect next. Lower the bed to avoid risk of falls, reapply any restraints, and raise the bedrails if needed. As you leave, clean your equipment, dispose of waste materials, and wash your hands.

The *General Survey* of the patient's build, height, and weight begins with the opening moments of the encounter. It is important to heighten the acuity of your clinical perceptions of the patient's mood, build, and behavior.

Nutritional status affects many characteristics you scrutinize during the *General Survey:* height, weight, blood pressure, posture, mood, alertness, facial coloration, dentition and condition of the tongue and gingiva, color of the nail beds, and muscle bulk. Be sure that assessments of height, weight, BMI, and risk of obesity are a routine part of your clinical practice.

Recapture observations you have been making since the first moments of your interaction. Sharpen them throughout.

TECHNIQUES	POSSIBLE FINDINGS

GENERAL SURVEY

Apparent State of Health	Acutely or chronically ill, frail, robust, vigorous
Level of Consciousness. Is the patient awake, alert, and interactive?	If not, promptly assess level of consciousness (see p. 270).
Signs of Distress ■ Cardiac or respiratory distress	Clutching the chest, pallor, diaphoresis; labored breathing, wheezing, cough
■ Pain	Wincing, sweating, protecting painful area
■ Anxiety or depression	Anxious face, fidgety movements, cold and moist palms; inexpressive or flat affect, poor eye contact, psychomotor slowing

TECHNIQUES	POSSIBLE FINDINGS
Height and Build **Weight**	Generalized fat in simple obesity; truncal fat with relatively thin limbs in Cushing's syndrome and syndrome X
Skin Color and Obvious Lesions. See Chapter 4, *The Skin, Hair, and Nails,* for details.	Pallor, cyanosis, jaundice, rashes, bruises
Dress, Grooming, and Personal Hygiene ■ Is the patient wearing any unusual jewelry? Where? Is there any body piercing? ■ Note patient's hair, fingernails, and use of cosmetics.	
Facial Expression. Watch for eye contact. Is it natural? Sustained and unblinking? Averted quickly? Absent?	Stare of hyperthyroidism; flat or sad affect of depression. Decreased eye contact may be cultural or may suggest anxiety, fear, or sadness.
Odors of Body and Breath. Odors can be important diagnostic clues, such as the fruity odor of diabetes or the scent of alcohol. Never assume that alcohol on a patient's breath explains changes in mental status or neurologic findings.	Breath odor of alcohol, acetone, uremia, or liver failure

TECHNIQUES	POSSIBLE FINDINGS

Posture, Gait, and Motor Activity

Preference to sit up in left-sided heart failure and to lean forward with arms braced in chronic obstructive pulmonary disease

VITAL SIGNS

Measure blood pressure, heart rate, respiratory rate, and temperature.

Blood Pressure. To measure blood pressure accurately, you must carefully choose a cuff of appropriate size.

SELECTING THE CORRECT BLOOD PRESSURE CUFF

- Width of the inflatable bladder of the cuff should be about 40% of upper arm circumference (about 12–14 cm in the average adult).
- Length of inflatable bladder should be about 80% of upper arm circumference (almost long enough to encircle the arm).
- If anaeroid, recalibrate periodically before use.

GETTING READY TO MEASURE BLOOD PRESSURE

- Ideally, ask the patient to avoid smoking or drinking caffeinated beverages for 30 minutes before the blood pressure is taken and to rest for at least 5 minutes.
- Check to make sure the examining room is quiet and comfortably warm.
- Make sure the arm selected is *free of clothing.* There should be no arteriovenous fistulas for dialysis, scarring from prior brachial artery cutdowns, or signs of lymphedema (seen after axillary node dissection or radiation therapy).

(continued)

GETTING READY TO MEASURE
BLOOD PRESSURE (Continued)

- Palpate the brachial artery to confirm that it has a viable pulse.
- Position the arm so that the brachial artery, at the antecubital crease, is *at heart level*—roughly level with the 4th interspace at its junction with the sternum.
- If the patient is seated, rest the arm on a table a little above the patient's waist; if standing, try to support the patient's arm at the midchest level.

MEASURING BLOOD PRESSURE

- Center the inflatable bladder over the brachial artery. The lower border of the cuff should be about 2.5 cm above the antecubital crease. Secure the cuff snugly. Position the patient's arm so that it is slightly flexed at the elbow.
- To determine how high to raise the cuff pressure, first estimate the systolic pressure by palpation. As you feel the radial artery with the fingers of one hand, rapidly inflate the cuff until the radial pulse disappears. Read this pressure on the manometer and add 30 mm Hg to it. Use of this sum as the target for subsequent inflations prevents discomfort from unnecessarily high cuff pressures. It also avoids the occasional error caused by an auscultatory gap—a silent interval between the systolic and diastolic pressures.
- Deflate the cuff promptly.
- Now place the bell of a stethoscope lightly over the brachial artery, taking care to make an air seal with its full rim. Because the sounds to be heard *(Korotkoff sounds)* are relatively low in pitch, they are heard better with the bell.
- Inflate the cuff rapidly again to the level just determined, and then deflate it slowly at a rate of about 2 to 3 mm Hg per second. Note the level at which you hear the sounds of at least two consecutive beats. This is the systolic pressure.

(continued)

TECHNIQUES	POSSIBLE FINDINGS

MEASURING BLOOD PRESSURE (Continued)

- Continue to lower the pressure slowly. The disappearance point, usually only a few mm Hg below the muffling point, enables the best estimate of true diastolic pressure in adults.
- Read both the systolic and diastolic levels to the nearest 2 mm Hg. Wait 2 or more minutes and repeat. Average your readings. If the first two readings differ by more than 5 mm Hg, take additional readings.
- Take blood pressure in both arms at least once.
- In patients taking antihypertensive medications or with a history of fainting, postural dizziness, or possible depletion of blood volume, take the blood pressure in three positions—supine, sitting, and standing (unless contraindicated).

In 1997, the Joint National Committee on Detection, Evaluation, and Treatment of High Blood Pressure categorized six levels of systolic blood pressure (SPB) and diastolic blood pressure (DPB):

A fall in systolic pressure of 20 mm Hg or more, especially when accompanied by symptoms, indicates orthostatic (postural) hypotension.

Blood Pressure Classification (Adults)*		
Category	Systolic (mm Hg)	Diastolic (mm Hg)
Hypertension		
Stage 3 (severe)	≥180	≥110
Stage 2 (moderate)	160–179	100–109
Stage 1 (mild)	140–159	90–99
High Normal	130–139	85–89
Normal	<130	<85
Optimal	<120	<80

*When the systolic and diastolic levels indicate different categories, use the higher category. For example, 170/92 mm Hg is moderate hypertension and 170/120 mm Hg is severe hypertension.

In *isolated systolic hypertension,* systolic pressure is 140 mm Hg or more and diastolic pressure is less than 90 mm Hg.

TECHNIQUES	POSSIBLE FINDINGS

Look for evidence of hypertensive retinopathy, left ventricular hypertrophy, and neurologic deficits suggesting a stroke.

Heart Rate. The radial pulse is used commonly to assess heart rate. With the pads of your index and middle fingers, compress the radial artery until you detect a maximal pulsation. If the rhythm is regular, count the rate for 15 seconds and multiply by 4. If the rate is unusually fast or slow, count it for 60 seconds. When the rhythm is irregular, evaluate the rate by auscultation at the cardiac apex (the apical pulse).

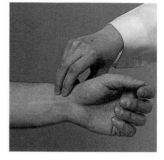

Heart Rhythm. Feel the radial pulse. Check the rhythm again by listening with your stethoscope at the cardiac apex. Is the rhythm regular or irregular? If irregular, try to identify a pattern: (1) Do early beats appear in a basically regular rhythm? (2) Does the irregularity vary consistently with respiration? (3) Is the rhythm totally irregular?

Palpation of an irregularly irregular rhythm reliably indicates *atrial fibrillation.* For all other irregular patterns, an ECG is needed to identify the arrhythmia. See Table 3-7, Rate and Rhythm of Breathing.

TECHNIQUES	POSSIBLE FINDINGS

Respiratory Rate and Rhythm. Observe the *rate, rhythm, depth,* and *effort of breathing.* Count the number of respirations in 1 minute either by visual inspection or by subtly listening over the patient's trachea with your stethoscope during your examination of the head and neck or chest. Normally, adults take 14 to 20 breaths per minute in a quiet, regular pattern.

See Table 3-7, Rate and Rhythm of Breathing.

Temperature. Average *oral temperature,* usually quoted at 37°C (98.6°F), fluctuates considerably from the early morning to the late afternoon or evening. *Rectal temperatures are higher* than oral temperatures by about 0.4 to 0.5°C (0.7 to 0.9°F), but this difference also varies. (In contrast, *axillary temperatures* are *lower* than oral temperatures by approximately 1°, but take 5 to 10 minutes to register and are considered less accurate than other measurements.)

Fever or pyrexia refers to an elevated body temperature. *Hyperpyrexia* refers to extreme elevation in temperature, above 41.1°C (106°F), while *hypothermia* refers to an abnormally low temperature, below 35°C (95°F) rectally.

TECHNIQUES	POSSIBLE FINDINGS

For *oral temperatures,* choose either a glass or electronic thermometer. When using a glass thermometer, shake the thermometer down to 35°C (96°F) or below, insert it under the tongue, instruct the patient to close both lips, and wait 3 to 5 minutes. Then read the thermometer, reinsert it for 1 minute, and read it again.

Causes of *fever* include infection, trauma (such as surgery or crush injuries), malignancy, blood disorders (such as acute hemolytic anemia), drug reactions, and immune disorders (such as collagen vascular disease).

If using an electronic thermometer, carefully place the disposable cover over the probe and insert the thermometer under the tongue. Accurate temperature recording usually takes about 10 seconds. Taking the *tympanic membrane temperature* is increasingly common and is quick, safe, and reliable if performed properly. Make sure the external auditory canal is free of cerumen. Position the probe in the canal. Wait 2 to 3 seconds until the digital temperature reading appears. This method measures core body temperature, which is higher than the normal oral temperature by approximately 0.8°C (1.4°F).

The chief cause of *hypothermia* is exposure to cold. Other predisposing causes include reduced movement as in paralysis, interference with vasoconstriction as from sepsis or excess alcohol, starvation, hypothyroidism, and hypoglycemia. Older adults are especially susceptible to hypothermia and also less likely to develop fever.

Recording the Physical Examination—General Survey and Vital Signs

Record the vital signs taken at the time of your examination. They are preferable to those taken earlier in the day by other providers. (Common abbreviations for blood pressure, heart rate, and respiratory rate are self-explanatory.)

"Mrs. Scott is a young, healthy-appearing woman, well-groomed, fit, and in good spirits. Height is 5′4″, weight 135 lbs, BP 120/80, HR 72 and regular, RR 16, temperature 37.5°C."

OR

"Mr. Jones is an elderly male who looks pale and chronically ill. He is alert, with good eye contact, but cannot speak more than two or three words at a time because of shortness of breath. He has intercostal muscle retraction when breathing and sits upright in bed. He is thin, with diffuse muscle wasting. Height is 6′2″, weight 175 lbs, BP 160/95, HR 108 and irregular, RR 32 and labored, temperature 101.2°F."

AIDS TO INTERPRETATION

TABLE 3-1 ■ Body Mass Index Chart

	19	20	21	22	23	24	25	26	27	28	29	30	31	32	33	34	35
Height (inches)							Body Weight (pounds)										
58	91	96	100	105	110	115	119	124	129	134	138	143	148	153	158	162	167
59	94	99	104	109	114	119	124	128	133	138	143	148	153	158	163	168	173
60	97	102	107	112	118	123	128	133	138	143	148	153	158	163	168	174	179
61	100	105	111	116	122	127	132	137	143	148	153	158	164	169	174	180	185
62	104	109	115	120	126	131	136	142	147	153	158	164	169	175	180	185	191
63	107	113	118	124	130	135	141	145	152	158	163	169	174	180	185	191	197
64	110	116	122	128	134	140	145	151	157	163	169	174	180	185	192	197	204
65	114	120	126	132	138	144	150	156	162	168	174	180	186	192	198	204	210
66	118	124	130	136	142	148	155	161	167	173	179	186	192	198	204	210	216
67	121	127	134	140	146	153	159	166	172	178	185	191	198	204	211	217	223
68	125	131	138	144	151	158	164	171	177	184	190	197	203	210	216	223	230
69	128	135	142	149	155	162	169	176	182	189	196	203	209	216	223	230	236
70	132	139	146	153	160	167	174	181	188	189	196	203	209	216	223	230	236
71	136	143	150	157	165	172	179	186	193	200	208	215	222	229	236	243	250
72	140	147	154	162	169	177	184	191	199	206	213	221	228	235	242	250	258
73	144	151	159	166	174	182	189	197	204	212	219	227	235	242	250	257	265
74	148	155	163	171	179	186	194	202	210	218	225	233	241	249	256	264	272
75	152	160	168	176	184	192	200	208	216	224	232	240	248	256	264	272	279
76	156	164	172	180	189	197	205	213	221	230	238	246	254	263	271	279	287

Source: Clinical Guidelines on the Identification, Evaluation, and Treatment of Overweight and Obesity in Adults, National Institutes of Health and National Heart, Lung and Blood Institute. June 1998.

TABLE 3-2 ■ Body Mass Index Nomogram: Adults

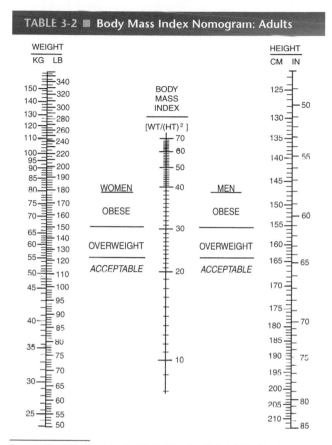

Source: Katz DL: Nutrition in Clinical Practice. Philadelphia, Lippincott Williams & Wilkins, 2001:340.

TABLE 3-3 ■ Eating Disorders and Excessively Low BMI

Anorexia Nervosa	Bulimia Nervosa
■ Refusal to maintain minimally normal body weight (or BMI above 17.5 kg/m²)	■ Repeated binge eating followed by self-induced vomiting, misuse of laxatives, diuretics or other medications, fasting; or excessive exercise
■ Fear of appearing fat	
■ Frequently starving but in denial; lacking insight	■ Overeating at least twice a week during 3-month period; large amounts of food consumed in short period (~2 hrs)
■ Often brought in by family members	
■ May present as failure to make expected weight gains in childhood or adolescence, amenorrhea in women, loss of libido or potency in men	■ Preoccupation with eating; craving and compulsion to eat; lack of control over eating; alternating with periods of starvation
■ Associated with depressive symptoms such as depressed mood, irritability, social withdrawal, insomnia, decreased libido	■ Dread of fatness but may be obese

■ Additional features supporting diagnosis: self-induced vomiting or purging, excessive exercise, use of appetite suppressants and/or diuretics	■ Subtypes of
	  ■ *Purging:* bulimic episodes accompanied by self-induced vomiting or use of laxatives, diuretics, or enemas
	  ■ *Nonpurging:* bulimic episodes accompanied by compensatory behavior such as fasting, exercise without purging

■ Biologic complications
  ■ *Neuroendocrine changes:* amenorrhea, hormonal alterations
  ■ *Cardiovascular disorders:* bradycardia, hypotension, dysrhythmias, cardiomyopathy
  ■ *Metabolic disorders:* hypokalemia, hypochloremic metabolic alkalosis, increased BUN, edema
  ■ *Other:* dry skin, dental caries, delayed gastric emptying, constipation, anemia, osteoporosis
	■ Biologic complications See changes listed for anorexia nervosa.

(Sources: World Health Organization: The ICD-10 Classification of Mental and Behavioral Disorders: Diagnostic Criteria for Research. World Health Organization, Geneva, 1993. American Psychiatric Association: DSM-IV-TR: Diagnostic and Statistical Manual of Mental Disorders, 4th ed. Text Revision. American Psychiatric Association, Washington, DC, 2000. Halmi, KA: Eating Disorders: In: Kaplan, HI, Sadock BJ, eds. Comprehensive Textbook of Psychiatry, 7th ed. Philadelphia, Lippincott Williams & Wilkins; 2000:1663–1676.)

TABLE 3-4 ■ Nutrition Counseling: Sources of Nutrients

Nutrient	Food Source
Calcium	Dairy foods such as yogurt, milk, and natural cheeses Breakfast cereal, fruit juice with calcium supplements Dark green leafy vegetables such as collards, turnip greens
Iron	Shellfish Lean meat, dark turkey meat Cereals with iron supplements Spinach, peas, lentils Enriched and whole-grain bread
Folate	Cooked dried beans and peas Oranges, orange juice Dark-green leafy vegetables
Vitamin D	Milk (fortified) Eggs, butter, margarine Cereals (fortified)

(Source: Adapted from Dietary Guidelines Committee, 2000 Report. "Nutrition and Your Health: Dietary Guidelines for Americans," Washington, DC, Agricultural Research Service, U.S. Department of Agriculture.)

TABLE 3-5 ■ Patients With Hypertension: Recommended Changes in Diet

Dietary Change	Food Source
Increase foods high in potassium	Baked white or sweet potatoes, cooked greens such as spinach Bananas, plantains, many dried fruits, orange juice
Decrease foods high in sodium	Canned foods (soups, tuna fish) Pretzels, potato chips, pickles, olives Many processed foods (frozen dinners, ketchup, mustard) Batter-fried foods Table salt, including for cooking

(Source: Adapted from Dietary Guidelines Committee, 2000 Report. "Nutrition and Your Health: Dietary Guidelines for Americans," Washington, DC, Agricultural Research Service, U.S. Department of Agriculture.)

TABLE 3-6 ■ Abnormalities of the Arterial Pulse and Pressure Waves

Normal. Pulse pressure is about 30 to 40 mm Hg. Pulse contour is smooth and rounded. (The notch on the descending slope of the pulse wave is not palpable.)

mm Hg

Small, weak pulses. Pulse pressure is diminished, and pulse feels weak and small. Upstroke may feel slowed, peak prolonged. Causes include (1) decreased stroke volume, as in heart failure, hypovolemia, and severe aortic stenosis, and (2) increased peripheral resistance, as in exposure to cold and severe congestive heart failure.

Large, bounding pulses. Pulse resistance is increased; pulse feels strong and bounding. Rise and fall may feel rapid, peak brief. Causes include (1) an increased stroke volume, a decreased peripheral resistance, or both, as in fever, anemia, hyperthyroidism, aortic regurgitation, arteriovenous fistulas, and patent ductus arteriosus, (2) an increased stroke volume from slow heart rates, as in bradycardia and complete heart block, and (3) decreased compliance (increased stiffness) of the aortic walls, as in aging or atherosclerosis.

Bisferient pulse. Arterial pulse is increased with a double systolic peak. Causes include pure aortic regurgitation, combined aortic stenosis and regurgitation, and, though less commonly palpable, hypertrophic cardiomyopathy.

(table continues next page)

TABLE 3-6 ■ Abnormalities of the Arterial Pulse and Pressure Waves *(Continued)*

Pulsus alterans. Pulse alternates in amplitude from beat to beat even though the rhythm is basically regular (and must be to make this judgment). When the difference between stronger and weaker beats is slight, only sphygmomanometry can detect it. Pulsus alterans indicates left ventricular failure and usually is accompanied by a left-sided S_3.

Bigeminal pulse. This rhythm disorder may masquerade as pulsus alterans. The cause is a normal beat alternating with a premature contraction. Stroke volume of the premature beat is diminished in relation to that of the normal beats. Pulse varies in amplitude accordingly.

Premature contractions

Paradoxical pulse. This may be detected by a palpable decrease in pulse's amplitude on quiet inspiration. If the sign is less pronounced, a blood-pressure cuff is needed. Systolic pressure decreases by more than 10 mm Hg during inspiration. It is found in precardial tamponade.

Expiration ← → Inspiration

TABLE 3-7 ■ Rate and Rhythm of Breathing

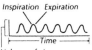

Inspiration Expiration

— Time —

Volume of air

Normal. In adults, 14 to 20 per minute; in infants, up to 44 per minute

Rapid Shallow Breathing (Tachypnea). Many causes, including restrictive lung disease, pleural chest pain, and an elevated diaphragm

Rapid Deep Breathing (Hyperpnea, hyperventilation). Many causes, including exercise, anxiety, metabolic acidosis, brainstem injury. *Kussmaul breathing,* due to metabolic acidosis, is deep but rate may be fast, slow, or normal.

Slow Breathing. May be secondary to diabetic coma, drug-induced respiratory depression, increased intracranial pressure

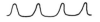
Hyperpnea   Apnea

Cheyne-Stokes Breathing. Rhythmically alternating periods of hyperpnea and apnea. In infants and the aged, may be normal during sleep; also accompanies brain damage, heart failure, uremia, drug-induced respiratory depression

Ataxic (Biot's) Breathing. Unpredictable irregularity of depth and rate. Causes include brain damage and respiratory depression

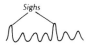
Sighs

Sighing Breathing. Breathing punctuated by frequent sighs. When associated with other symptoms, it suggests the hyperventilation syndrome. Occasional sighs are normal.

The Skin, Hair, and Nails

4

THE HEALTH HISTORY

Common or Concerning Symptoms

- Hair loss
- Rash
- Moles

HEALTH PROMOTION AND COUNSELING

Important Topics for Health Promotion and Counseling

- Risk factors for melanoma
- Avoidance of excessive sun exposure

Counsel patient to avoid unnecessary sun exposure and to use sunscreen with SPF-15. Teach ABCDE screen for dysplastic nevi/melanomas: **A**symmetry, irregular **B**orders, variation in **C**olor, **D**iameter >6 mm, **E**levation. Survey skin at 3-year intervals for patients 20 to 39 years of age and annually for patients older than 40 years.

TECHNIQUES	POSSIBLE FINDINGS

TECHNIQUES OF EXAMINATION

SKIN

Examine each region.
Inspect and **palpate**.

Note:

■ Color	Cyanosis, jaundice, carotenemia, changes in melanin
■ Moisture	Moist, dry, oily
■ Temperature	Cool, warm
■ Texture	Smooth, rough
■ Mobility—ease with which a fold of skin can be moved	Decreased in edema
■ Turgor—speed with which the fold returns into place	Decreased in dehydration

Note any lesions and their

■ Anatomic location	Generalized, localized
■ Arrangement	Linear, clustered, dermatomal
■ Type	Macule, papule, pustule, bulla, tumor
■ Color	Red, white, brown, mauve

TECHNIQUES	POSSIBLE FINDINGS

NAILS

Inspect and **palpate** the fingernails and toenails.

Note

■ Color	Cyanosis, pallor
■ Shape	Clubbing
■ Any lesions	Paronychia, onycholysis

HAIR

Inspect and **palpate** the hair.

Note

■ Quantity	Thin, thick
■ Distribution	Patchy or total alopecia
■ Texture	Fine, coarse

Recording the Physical Examination—
The Skin, Hair, and Nails

"Color good. Skin warm and moist. Nails without clubbing or cyanosis. No suspicious nevi, rash, petechiae, or ecchymoses."

AIDS TO INTERPRETATION

TABLE 4-1 ■ Color Changes in the Skin

Color/Mechanism	Selected Causes
Brown: Increased melanin (greater than a person's genetic norm)	Sun exposure Pregnancy (melasma) Addison's disease
Blue (cyanosis): Increased deoxyhemoglobin from hypoxia: ■ Peripheral ■ Central (arterial)	 Anxiety or cold environment Heart or lung disease
Abnormal hemoglobin	Methemoglobinemia, sulfhemoglobinemia
Red: Increased visibility of oxyhemoglobin from: ■ Dilated superficial blood vessels or increased blood flow in skin ■ Decreased use of oxygen in skin	 Fever, blushing, alcohol intake, local inflammation Cold exposure (e.g., cold ears)
Yellow: Increased bilirubin of jaundice (sclera looks yellow)	 Liver disease, hemolysis of red blood cells
Carotenemia (sclera does not look yellow)	Increased carotene intake from yellow fruits and vegetables
Pale: Decreased melanin	 Albinism, vitiligo, tinea versicolor
Decreased visibility of oxyhemoglobin from: ■ Decreased blood flow to skin ■ Decreased amount of oxyhemoglobin	 Syncope or shock Anemia
Edema (may mask skin pigments)	Nephrotic syndrome

TABLE 4-2 ■ Types of Skin Lesions

Primary Lesions

Circumscribed, flat, nonpalpable changes in color:

MACULE. Small spot. *Examples:* freckle, petechia

PATCH. Larger macule. *Example:* vitiligo

Palpable, elevated, solid masses:

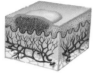

PAPULE. Up to 1 cm. *Example:* the papule of acne

PLAQUE. An elevated flat surface larger than 1 cm. *Example:* xanthelasma of the eyelids

NODULE. Larger than 0.5 cm; often deeper and firmer than a papule. *Example:* epidermoid cyst

TUMOR. Large nodule. *Example:* a large neurofibroma

WHEAL. A relatively transient, superficial area of local skin edema. *Example:* mosquito bite

Circumscribed superficial elevations of the skin formed by free fluid in a cavity between the skin layers:

VESICLE. Up to 0.5 cm; filled with serous fluid. *Example:* poison ivy

BULLA. Greater than 0.5 cm; filled with serous fluid. *Example:* 2nd-degree burn

PUSTULE. Filled with pus. *Example:* acne

(table continues next page)

TABLE 4-2 ■ Types of Skin Lesions *(Continued)*

Secondary Lesions

Loss of skin surface:

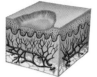

EROSION. Loss of superficial epidermis, leaving a moist area that does not bleed. *Example:* skin surface after a ruptured vesicle

ULCER. A deeper loss of surface that may bleed and scar. *Examples:* syphilitic chancre, ulcer of venous insufficiency

FISSURE. A linear crack. *Example:* athlete's foot

Material on the skin surface:

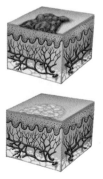

CRUST. The dried residue of serum, pus, or blood. *Example:* a scab

SCALE. A thin flake of exfoliated epidermis. *Examples:* dry skin, dandruff

TABLE 4-3 ■ Characteristics of Nevi (Moles)

Normal

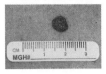

Diameter smaller than 6 millimeters
Symmetric; regular borders, even in color

Malignant Melanoma (ABCDE)

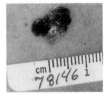

Asymmetric

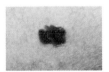

Borders irregular

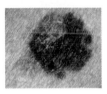

Color varied
Diameter more than 6 mm
Elevation

(Courtesy of American Cancer Society; American Academy of Dermatology)

TABLE 4-4 ■ Vascular and Purpuric Lesions of the Skin

Lesion	Features
Spider Angioma 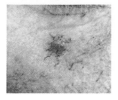	**Appearance:** Fiery red; very small to 2 cm; central body, sometimes raised, radiating with erythema **Distribution:** Face, neck, arms, and upper trunk, but almost never below the waist **Significance:** Liver disease, pregnancy, vitamin B deficiency; normal in some people
Spider Vein 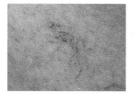	**Appearance:** Bluish; varies from very small to several inches; may resemble a spider or be linear, irregular, or cascading **Distribution:** Most often on the legs, near veins; also on anterior chest **Significance:** Often accompanies increased pressure in the superficial veins, as in varicose veins
Cherry Angioma 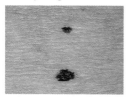	**Appearance:** Bright or ruby red, may become brownish with age; 1–3 mm; round, flat, sometimes raised; may be surrounded by a pale halo **Distribution:** Found on trunk or extremities **Significance:** None; increase in size and number with aging

(table continues next page)

TABLE 4-4 ■ Vascular and Purpuric Lesions of the Skin (Continued)

Lesion	Features
Petechia and Purpura 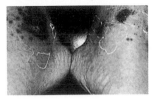	**Appearance:** Deep red or reddish purple; fades over time; 1–3 mm or larger; rounded, sometimes irregular, flat **Distribution:** Varies **Significance:** Blood outside the vessels; may suggest a bleeding disorder or, if petechiae, emboli to skin
Ecchymosis 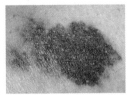	**Appearance:** Purple or purplish blue, fading to green, yellow, and brown over time; larger than petechiae; rounded, oval, or irregular **Distribution:** Varies **Significance:** Blood outside the vessels; often secondary to bruising or trauma; also seen in bleeding disorders

TABLE 4-5 ■ Skin Tumors

Actinic Keratoses are superficial, flattened papules covered by a dry scale. Often multiple, they may be round or irregular, and are pink, tan, or grayish. They appear on sun-exposed skin of older, fair-skinned persons. Though themselves benign, these lesions may give rise to squamous cell carcinoma (suggested by rapid growth, induration, redness at the base, and ulceration). Typical locations are face and hands.

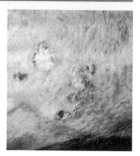

Seborrheic Keratoses are common, benign, yellowish to brown, raised lesions that feel slightly greasy and velvety or warty. Typically multiple and symmetrically distributed on the trunk of older people, they may also appear on the face and elsewhere. In blacks, they may appear as small, deeply pigmented papules on the cheeks and temples (dermatosis papulosa nigra).

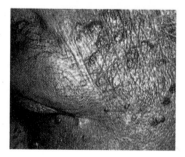

(table continues next page)

TABLE 4-5 ■ Skin Tumors *(Continued)*

Basal Cell Carcinoma, though malignant, grows slowly and seldom metastasizes. It is most common in fair-skinned adults older than age 40, and usually appears on the face. An initial translucent nodule spreads, leaving a depressed center and a firm, elevated border. Telangiectatic vessels are often visible.

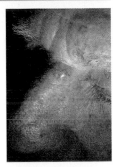

Squamous Cell Carcinoma usually appears on sun-exposed skin of fair-skinned adults older than 60. It may develop in an actinic keratosis. It usually grows more quickly than a basal cell carcinoma, is firmer, and looks redder. The face and the back of the hand are often affected.

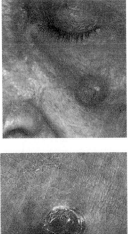

Kaposi's Sarcoma in AIDS may appear in many forms: macules, papules, plaques, or nodules almost anywhere on the body. Lesions are often multiple and may involve internal structures.

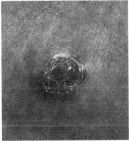

TABLE 4-6 ■ Fingernails

Clubbing

Dorsal phalanx rounded and bulbous; convexity of nail plate increased. Angle between plate and proximal nail fold increased to 180° or more. Proximal nail folds feel spongy. Many causes, including chronic hypoxia and lung cancer

Paronychia

Inflammation of proximal and lateral nail folds, acute or chronic. Folds red, swollen, may be tender.

Onycholysis

Painless separation of nail plate from nail bed, starting distally. Many causes.

Terry's Nails

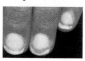

Whitish with a distal band of reddish brown. Seen in aging and some chronic diseases.

Leukonychia

White spots caused by trauma. They grow out with nail(s).

Transverse White Lines

Curved white lines similar to curve of lunula. They follow an illness and grow out with nails.

The Head and Neck

5

THE HEALTH HISTORY

Common or Concerning Symptoms

- Headache
- Change in vision
- Double vision, or diplopia
- Hearing loss, earache; tinnitus
- Vertigo
- Nosebleed, or epistaxis
- Sore throat; hoarseness
- Swollen glands
- Goiter

THE HEAD

Headache is an extremely common symptom that always requires careful evaluation because a small fraction of headaches arise from life-threatening conditions. Elicit a full description of the headache and all seven attributes of the patient's pain (see p. 22).

See Table 5-1, Headaches, pp. 84–88. Tension and migraine headaches are the most common recurring headaches.

Is the headache one-sided or bilateral? Steady or throbbing? Continuous or comes and goes? Ask the patient to *point to the area of pain or discomfort.* Assess *chronologic pattern* and *severity.*

Tension headaches often arise in the temporal areas; cluster headaches may be retro-orbital.

Changing or progressively severe headaches increase the likelihood of tumor, abscess, or other mass lesion. Extremely severe headaches suggest subarachnoid hemorrhage or meningitis.

Ask about associated symptoms. Inquire specifically about associated nausea and vomiting and neurologic symptoms such as change in vision or motor-sensory deficits.

Visual aura or scintillating scotomas may accompany migraine. Nausea and vomiting are common with migraine but also occur with brain tumor and subarachnoid hemorrhage.

Ask whether coughing, sneezing, or changing the position of the head has any effect (better, worse, or none) on the headache.

Such maneuvers may increase pain from brain tumor and acute sinusitis.

Ask about family history.

Family history may be positive in patients with migraine.

THE EYES

Ask "How is your vision?" and "Have you had any trouble with your eyes?" If the patient reports a change in vision, pursue the related details:

Refractive errors often explain gradual blurring. High blood glucose levels may cause blurring.

■ Is the onset sudden or gradual?	Sudden visual loss suggests retinal detachment, vitreous hemorrhage, or occlusion of the central retinal artery.
■ Is the problem worse during close work or at distances?	Difficulty with close work suggests *hyperopia* (farsightedness) or *presbyopia* (aging vision); difficulty with distances suggests *myopia* (near-sightedness).
■ Is there blurring of the entire field of vision or only parts? Is blurring central, peripheral, or only on one side?	Slow central loss in *nuclear cataract* and macular *degeneration*; peripheral loss in advanced *open-angle glaucoma*; one-sided loss in *hemianopsia* and quadrantic defects (p. 75).
■ Has the patient seen lights flashing across the field of vision? Vitreous floaters?	Flashing lights or new vitreous floaters suggest detachment of vitreous from retina. Prompt eye consultation is indicated.
Ask about *pain* in or around the eyes, *redness,* and *excessive tearing* or *watering*.	
Check for *diplopia,* or double vision.	Diplopia may arise from a lesion in the brainstem or cerebellum or from weakness or paralysis of one or more extraocular muscles.

THE EARS

Ask "How is your hearing?"	See Table 5-7, Patterns of Hearing Loss, p. 95.

Does the patient have special difficulty understanding people as they talk? What difference does a noisy environment make?

People with sensorineural loss have particular trouble understanding speech, often complaining that others mumble; noisy environments worsen hearing. In conductive loss, noisy environments may help.

For complaints of *earache,* or *pain in the ear,* ask about associated fever, sore throat, cough, and concurrent upper respiratory infection.

For pain in the external ear, consider *otitis externa;* for pain associated with respiratory infection and in the inner ear, consider *otitis media.*

Tinnitus has no external stimulus—commonly, it manifests as a musical ringing or a rushing or roaring noise.

When associated with hearing loss and vertigo, tinnitus suggests Ménière's disease.

Ask about *vertigo,* the perception that the patient or the environment is rotating or spinning.

THE NOSE AND SINUSES

Rhinorrhea, or drainage from the nose, frequently is associated with *nasal congestion,* a sense of stuffiness or obstruction. Ask further about *sneezing,* watery eyes, and throat discomfort, and also *itching* in the eyes, nose, and throat.

Causes include viral infections, allergic rhinitis ("hay fever"), and vasomotor rhinitis. Itching favors an allergic cause.

For *epistaxis,* or bleeding from the nose, identify the source carefully—is bleeding from the nose or has the patient coughed up or vomited blood? Assess the site of bleeding, its severity, and associated symptoms.

Local causes of epistaxis include trauma (especially nose picking), inflammation, drying and crusting of the nasal mucosa, tumors, and foreign bodies.

THE MOUTH, THROAT, AND NECK

Sore throat is a frequent complaint. Ask about fever, swollen glands, and any associated cough.

Fever, pharyngeal exudates, and anterior cervical lymphadenopathy, especially without cough, suggest streptococcal pharyngitis, or *strep throat* (p. 99).

Hoarseness may arise from laryngeal disease or when extrapharyngeal lesions press on the laryngeal nerves.

Assess thyroid function. Ask about *goiter, temperature intolerance,* and *sweating.*

With goiter, thyroid function may be increased, decreased, or normal. Cold intolerance suggests *hypothyroidism*; heat intolerance, palpitations, and involuntary weight loss suggest *hyperthyroidism* (p. 99).

HEALTH PROMOTION AND COUNSELING

Important Topics for Health Promotion and Counseling

- Changes in vision, cataracts, macular degeneration, glaucoma
- Hearing loss
- Oral health

Disorders of vision shift with age. Healthy young adults generally have refractive errors. Up to 25% of adults older than 65 years have refractive errors; however, *cataracts, macular degeneration,* and *glaucoma* become more prevalent. Glaucoma is the leading cause of blindness in African Americans and the second leading cause of blindness overall. Glaucoma causes gradual vision loss, with damage to the optic nerve, loss of visual fields, beginning usually at the periphery, and pallor and increasing size of the optic cup (enlarging to more than half the diameter of the optic disc).

More than one third of adults older than 65 years have *detectable hearing deficits.* Questionnaires and handheld audioscopes work well for periodic screening.

Be sure to promote *oral health:* up to half of all children 5 to 17 years of age have one to eight cavities, and the average U.S. adult has 10 to 17 decayed, missing, or filled teeth. More than half of all adults older than 65 years have no teeth! Inspect the oral cavity for decayed or loose teeth, inflammation of the gingiva, and signs of periodontal disease (bleeding, pus, receding gums, and bad breath). Counsel patients to use fluoride-containing toothpastes, brush, floss, and seek dental care at least annually.

TECHNIQUES	POSSIBLE FINDINGS

TECHNIQUES OF EXAMINATION

THE HEAD

Examine the

■ Hair, including quantity, distribution, and texture	Coarse and sparse in myxedema, fine in hyperthyroidism
■ Scalp, including lumps or lesions	Pilar cysts, psoriasis
■ Skull, including size and contour	Hydrocephalus, skull depression from trauma
■ Face, including symmetry and facial expression	Facial paralysis; flat affect of depression, moods such as anger, sadness
■ Skin, including color, texture, hair distribution, and lesions	Pale, fine, hirsute, acne, skin cancer

THE EYES

Test visual acuity in each eye.	Diminished acuity
Assess visual fields, if indicated.	Hemianopsia, quadrantic defects

Inspect the

■ Position and alignment of eyes	Exophthalmos, strabismus
■ Eyebrows	Seborrheic dermatitis
■ Eyelids	Sty, chalazion, ectropion, ptosis, xanthelasma

TECHNIQUES	POSSIBLE FINDINGS
■ Lacrimal apparatus	Swollen lacrimal sac
■ Conjunctiva and sclera	Red eye, jaundice
■ Cornea, iris, and lens	Corneal opacity, cataract
Examine pupils for	
■ Size, shape, and symmetry	Miosis, mydriasis, anisocoria
■ Reactions to light and if these are abnormal	Absent in paralysis of CN III
■ The near reaction	Useful in tonic and Argyll Robertson pupils

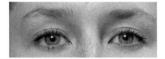 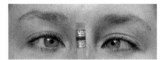

THE NEAR REACTION

Assess the extraocular muscles by observing

■ The corneal reflections from a midline light	Muscular imbalance
■ The six cardinal directions of gaze	Paralytic or nonparalytic strabismus, nystagmus, lid lag

Superior rectus (III)   Inferior oblique (III)   Superior rectus (III)
Lateral rectus (VI)   Medial rectus (III)   Lateral rectus (VI)
Inferior rectus (III)   Superior oblique (IV)   Inferior rectus (III)

■ Convergence	Poor in hyperthyroidism

TECHNIQUES	**POSSIBLE FINDINGS**

Inspect the fundi with an ophthalmoscope, including the

■ Red reflex

Cataracts, artificial eye

■ Optic disc

Papilledema, glaucomatous cupping, optic atrophy
See Table 5-4, Abnormalities of the Optic Disc, p. 92.

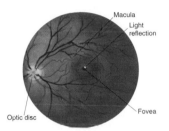

Macula
Light reflection
Fovea
Optic disc

From Tasman W, Jaeger E (eds): The Wills Eye Hospital Atlas of Clinical Ophthalmology, 2nd ed. Philadelphia, Lippincott Williams & Wilkins, 2001.

■ Arteries, veins, and A–V crossings

Hypertensive changes

■ Adjacent retina (note any lesions)

Hemorrhages, exudates, cotton-wool patches, microaneurysms, pigmentation

■ Macular area

Macular degeneration

■ Anterior structures

Vitreous floaters, cataracts

TECHNIQUES	POSSIBLE FINDINGS

TIPS FOR USING THE OPHTHALMOSCOPE

- Darken the room. Turn the lens disc to the large round beam of white light. *Lower the brightness of the light beam* to make the examination more comfortable for the patient.
- Turn the lens disc to the 0 diopter (a diopter measures the power of a lens to converge or diverge light).
- Hold the ophthalmoscope *in your right hand* to examine *the patient's right eye;* hold it *in your left hand* to examine *the patient's left eye* to avoid bumping the patient's nose.
- Hold the ophthalmoscope firmly braced against the medial aspect of your bony orbit, with the handle tilted laterally at about 20°. Instruct the patient to look slightly up and over your shoulder at a point directly ahead on the wall.
- Place yourself about 15 inches away from the patient and *at an angle 15° lateral to the patient's line of vision.* Look for the orange glow in the pupil—the *red reflex.* Note any opacities interrupting the red reflex. No red reflex suggests an opacity of the lens (cataract) or possibly the vitreous.
- Place the thumb of your other hand across the patient's eyebrow. Keeping the light beam focused on the red reflex, move in at a 15° angle toward the pupil until you almost touch the patient's eyelashes.

THE EARS

Examine on each side:

THE AURICLE

Inspect it.	Keloid, epidermoid cyst

If you suspect otitis:

■ Move the auricle up and down, and press on the tragus.	Pain in otitis externa
■ Press firmly behind the ear.	Possible tenderness in otitis media and mastoiditis

TIPS FOR EXAMINING THE OPTIC DISC AND THE RETINA

- *Locate the optic disc.* Look for the round yellowish-orange structure.
- Now, *bring the optic disc into sharp focus* by adjusting the lens of your ophthalmoscope.
- *Inspect the optic disc.* Note the following features:
  - *The sharpness or clarity of the disc outline*
  - *The color of the disc*
  - *The size of the physiologic cup* (an enlarged cup suggests chronic open-angle glaucoma)
  - *Venous pulsations* in the retinal veins as they emerge from the central portion of the disc (loss of venous pulsations in pathologic conditions such as head trauma, meningitis, or mass lesions may be an early sign of elevated intracranial pressure)
- *Inspect the retina.* Distinguish arteries from veins based on the features listed below.

	Arteries	Veins
Color	Light red	Dark red
Size	Smaller ($\frac{2}{3}$ to $\frac{4}{5}$ the diameter of veins)	Larger
Light Reflex (reflection)	Bright	Inconspicuous or absent

- *Follow the vessels peripherally in each of four directions.*
- Inspect the *fovea* and surrounding *macula.* Macular degeneration types include *dry atrophic* (more common but less severe) and *wet exudative* (neovascular). Undigested cellular debris, called *drusen,* may be hard or soft.
- Assess *papilledema.*

THE EAR CANAL AND EARDRUM

Pull the auricle up, back, and slightly out.

Inspect, through an otoscope speculum:

TECHNIQUES	POSSIBLE FINDINGS
■ The canal	Cerumen, otitis externa
■ The eardrum	Acute otitis media, serous otitis media, tympanosclerosis, perforations. See Table 5-6, Abnormal Eardrums, p. 94.

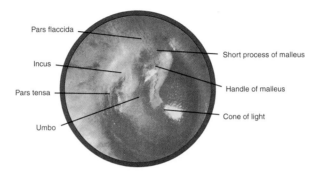

Pars flaccida

Incus

Pars tensa

Umbo

Short process of malleus

Handle of malleus

Cone of light

HEARING

Assess auditory acuity to whispered or spoken voice.

If hearing is diminished, use a 512-Hz tuning fork to

These tests help distinguish between sensorineural and conduction hearing loss.

■ Test lateralization (**Weber test**). Place vibrating and tuning fork on vertex of skull and check hearing.

■ Compare air and bone conduction (**Rinne test**). Place vibrating and tuning fork on mastoid bone, then remove and check hearing.

TECHNIQUES	POSSIBLE FINDINGS

THE NOSE AND SINUSES

Inspect the external nose.

Inspect, through a speculum, the

■ Nasal mucosa that covers the septum and turbinates, noting its color and any swelling	Swollen and red in viral rhinitis, swollen and pale in allergic rhinitis; polyps; ulcer from cocaine use
■ Nasal septum for position and integrity	Deviation, perforation
Palpate the frontal and maxillary sinuses for tenderness.	Tender in acute sinusitis

THE MOUTH AND PHARYNX

Inspect the

■ Lips	Cyanosis, pallor, cheilosis
■ Oral mucosa	Canker sores
■ Gums	Gingivitis, periodontal disease
■ Teeth	Dental caries, tooth loss
■ Roof of the mouth	Torus palatinus
■ Tongue, including	See Table 5-9, Tongues, pp. 97–98
Papillae	Glossitis
Symmetry	Paralysis of Cranial Nerve XII
Any lesions	Cancer

TECHNIQUES	POSSIBLE FINDINGS
■ Floor of the mouth	Cancer
■ Pharynx, including	See Table 5-10, Abnormalities of the Pharynx, p. 99.
Color or any exudate	Pharyngitis
Presence and size of tonsils	Tonsillitis, peritonsillar abscess
Symmetry of the soft palate as patient says "ah"	Paralysis of Cranial Nerve X

THE NECK

Inspect the neck.	Scars, masses, torticollis
Palpate the lymph nodes.	Cervical lymphadenopathy resulting from inflammation, malignancy
Inspect and **palpate** the position of the trachea.	Deviated trachea
Inspect the thyroid gland:	
■ At rest	Goiter, nodules
■ As patient swallows water	
From behind patient, **palpate** the thyroid gland, including the isthmus and the lateral lobes:	Goiter, nodules, tenderness of thyroiditis
■ At rest	
■ As patient swallows water	

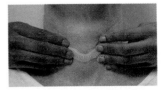

TECHNIQUES	POSSIBLE FINDINGS

You may conduct the initial survey of respiration during examination of the front of the neck. After feeling the thyroid gland from behind, you may proceed to a musculoskeletal examination of the neck and upper back and a check for costovertebral angle tenderness.

Recording the Physical Examination—The Head, Eyes, Ears, Nose, and Throat (HEENT)

HEENT: Head—Skull is normocephalic/atraumatic (NC/AT). Hair with average texture. *Eyes*—Visual acuity 20/20 bilaterally. Sclera white; conjunctiva pink. Pupils constrict 4 mm to 2 mm, equally round and reactive to light and accommodations. Disc margins sharp; no hemorrhages or exudates; no arteriolar narrowing. *Ears*—Acuity good to whispered voice. Tympanic membranes (TMs) with good cone of light. Weber midline. AC > BC. *Nose*—Nasal mucosa pink, septum midline; no sinus tenderness. *Throat (or Mouth)*—Oral mucosa pink; dentition good; pharynx without exudates. *Neck*—Trachea midline. Neck supple; thyroid isthmus palpable, lobes not felt. *Lymph Nodes*—No cervical, axillary, epitrochlear, inguinal adenopathy.

AIDS TO INTERPRETATION

TABLE 5-1 ■ Headaches

Problem	Common Characteristics	Associated Symptoms with Provoking and Relieving Factors
Tension Headaches	**Location:** Usually bilateral, may be generalized or localized to back of head and upper neck or to frontotemporal area **Quality:** Mild and aching or nonpainful tightness and pressure **Onset:** Gradual **Duration:** Varies hours to days, but often weeks or months	Anxiety, tension, depression ↑ by sustained muscular tension (driving, typing), emotions ↓ possibly by massage, relaxation
Migraine Headaches (*visual or neurologic symptoms 30 min before the headache distinguish "classic" from "common" migraine.*)	**Location:** Typically frontal or temporal, one or both sides, but also may be occipital or generalized; classic migraine typically unilateral **Quality:** Throbbing or aching; variable severity **Onset:** Fairly rapid, peaking in 1 to 2 hours	Often nausea and vomiting; some patients have preceding visual disturbances (local flashes of light, blind spots) or neurologic symptoms (local weakness, sensory disturbances, other symptoms) ↑ by alcohol, certain foods, tension, noise and bright light and before menses

(table continues next page)

TABLE 5-1 ■ Headaches *(Continued)*

Problem	Common Characteristics	Associated Symptoms with Provoking and Relieving Factors
	Duration: Several hours to 1 to 2 days	↓ by quiet, dark room; sleep; transient relief from pressure on the involved artery, if early in the course
Toxic Vascular Headaches (*resulting from fever, toxic substances, or drug withdrawal*)	**Location:** Generalized **Quality:** Aching; variable severity **Onset:** Variable **Duration:** Depends on cause	Depends on cause ↑ by fever, carbon monoxide, hypoxia, caffeine withdrawal
Cluster Headaches	**Location:** One-sided, high in the nose, and behind and over the eye **Quality:** Steady; severe **Onset:** Abrupt, often 2 to 3 hours after falling asleep **Duration:** Roughly 1 to 2 hours	Unilateral stuffy, runny nose and reddening and tearing of the eye During a cluster, may be provoked by alcohol
Headaches With Eye Disorders		
Errors of Refraction (*hyperopia and astigmatism, but not myopia*)	**Location:** Around and over the eyes; may radiate to occipital area **Quality:** Steady, aching, dull **Onset:** Gradual **Duration:** Variable	Eye fatigue, "sandy" sensations in the eyes, redness of the conjunctiva ↑ by prolonged use of the eyes, particularly for close work ↓ by resting the eyes

(table continues next page)

TABLE 5-1 ■ Headaches *(Continued)*

Problem	Common Characteristics	Associated Symptoms with Provoking and Relieving Factors
Acute Glaucoma	**Location:** In and around one eye **Quality:** Steady and aching; often severe **Onset:** Often rapid **Duration:** Variable; may depend on treatment	Diminished vision, sometimes nausea and vomiting ↑ sometimes by drops that dilate the pupils
Headaches with Acute Paranasal Sinusitis	**Location:** Usually above the eye (frontal sinus) or in the cheekbone area (maxillary sinus); one or both sides **Quality:** Aching or throbbing; variable severity **Onset:** Variable **Duration:** Often several hours at a time, recurring over days or longer	Local tenderness, nasal congestion, discharge, fever ↑ possibly by coughing, sneezing, or jarring the head ↓ by nasal decongestants
Trigeminal Neuralgia	**Location:** Cheeks, jaws, lips, or gums (2nd and 3rd divisions of trigeminal nerve) **Quality:** Sharp, short, brief, lightninglike jabs; very severe	Exhaustion from recurrent pain ↑ typically by touching certain areas of the lower face or mouth, chewing, talking, or brushing teeth

(table continues next page)

TABLE 5-1 ■ Headaches (Continued)

Problem	Common Characteristics	Associated Symptoms with Provoking and Relieving Factors
	Onset: Abrupt **Duration:** Each jab transient, but jabs recur in clusters at intervals of seconds or minutes	
Giant Cell Arteritis	**Location:** Localized near the involved artery (most often the temporal, also the occipital); may become generalized **Quality:** Aching, throbbing, or burning; often severe **Onset:** Gradual or rapid **Duration:** Variable	Tenderness of adjacent scalp, fever, malaise, fatigue, anorexia, muscular aches and stiffness, visual loss or blindness
Chronic Subdural Hematoma	**Location:** Variable **Quality:** Steady, aching **Onset:** Gradual, weeks to months after the injury **Duration:** Often depends on surgical intervention	Alterations in consciousness, personality changes, hemiparesis (weakness on one side of body); injury often forgotten

(table continues next page)

TABLE 5-1 ■ Headaches *(Continued)*

Problem	Common Characteristics	Associated Symptoms with Provoking and Relieving Factors
Post-concussion Syndrome	**Location:** Possibly, but not necessarily, localized to injured area **Quality:** Variable **Onset:** Within a few hours of the injury **Duration:** Weeks, months, or even years	Poor concentration, giddiness or vertigo, irritability, restlessness, tenseness, fatigue ↑ by mental and physical exertion, straining, stooping, emotional excitement, alcohol ↓ by rest
Meningitis	**Location:** Generalized **Quality:** Steady or throbbing; very severe **Onset:** Fairly rapid **Duration:** Variable, usually days	Fever, stiff neck
Subarachnoid Hemorrhage	**Location:** Generalized **Quality:** Very severe, "worst of my life" **Onset:** Usually abrupt; possible prodromal symptoms **Duration:** Variable, usually days	Nausea, vomiting, possible loss of consciousness, neck pain
Brain Tumor	**Location:** Varies **Quality:** Aching, steady; variable intensity **Onset:** Variable **Duration:** Often brief	Neurologic and mental symptoms, nausea and vomiting ↑ possibly by coughing, sneezing, or sudden movements of the head

TABLE 5-2 ■ Visual Field Defects

Altitudinal (horizontal) defect, usually resulting from a vascular lesion of the retina

Unilateral blindness, from a lesion of the retina or optic nerve

Bitemporal hemianopsia, from a lesion of the optic chiasm

Homonymous hemianopsia, from a lesion of the optic tract or optic radiation on the side opposite the blind area

Homonymous quadrantic defect, from a partial lesion of the optic radiation on the side opposite the blind area

LEFT   RIGHT

(*from patient's viewpoint*)

TABLE 5-3 ■ Physical Findings in and Around the Eye

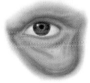

Herniated fat. A common cause of swelling in the lower lid and the inner third of the upper lid; associated with aging

Periorbital edema. Swelling of the eyelids from excessive fluid; many causes, including cellulitis, nephrotic syndrome

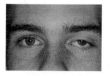

Ptosis. A drooping upper eyelid that narrows the palpebral fissure from a muscle or nerve disorder

(*table continues next page*)

TABLE 5-3 ■ Physical Findings in and Around the Eye *(Continued)*

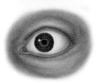
Enlarged palpebral fissure. Seen in retraction of the eyelids, exophthalmos, both signs of hyperthyroidism

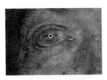
Ectropion. Outward turning of the margin of the lower lid, exposing the palpebral conjunctiva

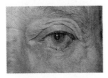
Entropion. Inward turning of the lid margin, causing irritation of the cornea or conjunctiva

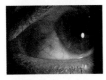
Pinguecula. Harmless yellowish nodule in the bulbar conjunctiva on either side of the iris; associated with aging

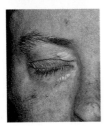
Xanthelasma. Yellowish plaques in the eyelids that may be caused by a lipid disorder

(table continues next page)

TABLE 5-3 ■ Physical Findings in and Around the Eye (Continued)

Basal cell epithelioma. A common skin cancer

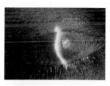

Chalazion. A beady nodule in either eyelid caused by a chronically inflamed meibomian gland

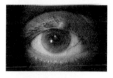

Sty. A pimplelike infection around a hair follicle near the lid margin

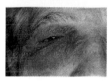

Dacryocystitis. An inflammation of the lacrimal sac, acute or chronic, that may obstruct tear drainage

Corneal arcus. A grayish white arc or ring often associated with aging

Pterygium. A thickening of the bulbar conjunctiva that may grow across the cornea

TABLE 5-4 ■ Abnormalities of the Optic Disc

	Process	Appearance
Normal	Tiny disc vessels give normal color to the disc.	Color is yellowish orange to creamy pink. Disc vessels are tiny. Disc margins are sharp (except perhaps nasally).
Optic atrophy	Death of optic nerve fibers leads to loss of the tiny disc vessels.	Color is white. Disc vessels are absent.
Papilledema	Venous stasis leads to engorgement and swelling.	Color is pink, hyperemic. Disc vessels are more visible, more numerous, and curve over the borders of the disc. Disc is swollen with margins blurred.
Glaucomatous cupping	Increased pressure within the eye leads to increased cupping (backward depression of the disc) and atrophy.	The base of the enlarged cup is pale.

TABLE 5-5 ∎ Diabetic Retinopathy

Nonproliferative Retinopathy, Moderately Severe

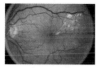

Note tiny red dots or microaneurysms. Note also the ring of hard exudates (white spots) located superotemporally. Retinal thickening or edema in the area of the hard exudates can impair visual acuity if it extends into the center of the macula (detection requires specialized stereoscopic examination).

Nonproliferative Retinopathy, Severe

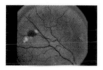

In the superior temporal quadrant, note the large retinal hemorrhage between two cotton-wool patches, beading of the retinal vein (just above them), and tiny tortuous retinal vessels above the superior temporal artery (termed *intraretinal micro-vascular abnormalities*).

Proliferative Retinopathy, with Neovascularization

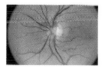

Note new preretinal vessels arising on the disc and extending across the disc margins. Visual acuity is currently normal, but risk of severe visual loss is high. (Photocoagulation can reduce this risk more than 50%.)

Proliferative Retinopathy, Advanced

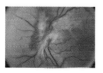

Same eye as above, but 2 years later and without treatment. Neovascularization has increased, now with fibrous proliferations, distortion of the macula, and reduced visual acuity.

(Source: Early Treatment Diabetic Retinopathy Study Research Group. Courtesy of M. F. Davis, MD, University of Wisconsin, Madison.)

TABLE 5-6 ■ Abnormal Eardrums

Serous Effusion

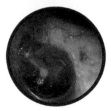

Amber fluid behind the eardrum, with or without air bubbles
Associated with viral upper respiratory infections or sudden changes in atmospheric pressure (diving, flying)

Acute Otitis Media

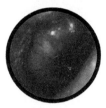

Red, bulging drum, loss of landmarks
Associated with bacterial infection

Tympanosclerosis

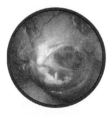

A chalky white patch
Scar of an old otitis media; of little or no clinical consequence

Perforation

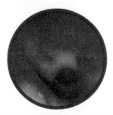

Hole in the eardrum that may be central or marginal
Usually the result of otitis media or trauma

TABLE 5-7 ■ Patterns of Hearing Loss

	Conductive Loss	Sensorineural Loss
Impaired understanding of words	Minor	Often troublesome
Effect of noisy environment	May help	Increases the hearing difficulty
Usual age of onset	Childhood, young adulthood	Middle and old age
Ear canal and drum	Often a visible abnormality	Problem not visible
Weber test (in unilateral hearing loss)	Lateralizes to the impaired ear	Lateralizes to the good ear
Rinne test	BC > AC or BC = AC	AC > BC
Causes include	Plugged ear canal, otitis media, immobile or perforated drum, otosclerosis	Sustained loud noise, drugs, inner ear infections, trauma, hereditary disorder, aging

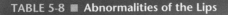

TABLE 5-8 ■ Abnormalities of the Lips

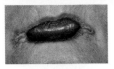

Angular cheilitis. Softening and cracking of the angles of the mouth

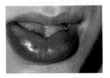

Angioedema. Diffuse, tense, subcutaneous swelling, usually allergic in cause

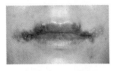

Herpes simplex. Painful vesicles, followed by crusting; also called **cold sore** or **fever blister**

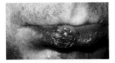

Syphilitic chancre. A firm lesion that ulcerates and may crust

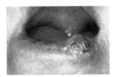

Carcinoma of the lip. A thickened plaque or irregular nodule that may ulcerate or crust; malignant

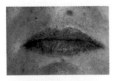

Hereditary hemorrhagic telangiectasia. Red spots, significant because of associated bleeding from nose and GI tract

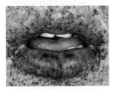

Peutz-Jeghers syndrome. Brown spots of the lips and buccal mucosa, significant because of their association with intestinal polyposis

TABLE 5-9 ■ Tongues

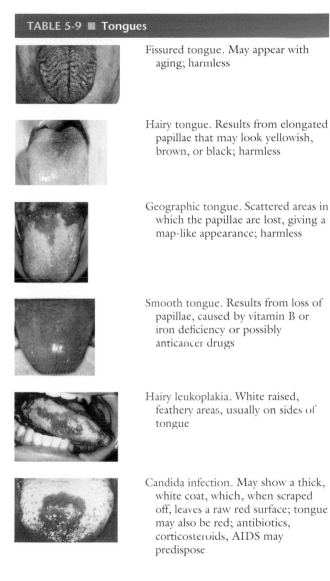

Fissured tongue. May appear with aging; harmless

Hairy tongue. Results from elongated papillae that may look yellowish, brown, or black; harmless

Geographic tongue. Scattered areas in which the papillae are lost, giving a map-like appearance; harmless

Smooth tongue. Results from loss of papillae, caused by vitamin B or iron deficiency or possibly anticancer drugs

Hairy leukoplakia. White raised, feathery areas, usually on sides of tongue

Candida infection. May show a thick, white coat, which, when scraped off, leaves a raw red surface; tongue may also be red; antibiotics, corticosteroids, AIDS may predispose

(table continues next page)

TABLE 5-9 ■ Tongues *(Continued)*

 Varicose veins. Dark round spots in the undersurface of the tongue, associated with aging; also called **caviar lesions**

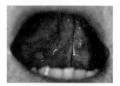 Aphthous ulcer (canker sore). Painful small, whitish ulcer with a red halo; heals in 7 to 10 days

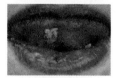 Mucous patch of syphilis. Slightly raised, oval lesion, covered by a grayish membrane

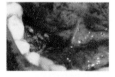 Carcinoma of the tongue or floor of the mouth. A malignancy that should be considered in any nodule or nonhealing ulcer at the base or edges of the mouth

TABLE 5-10 ■ Abnormalities of the Pharynx

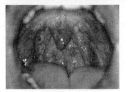

Pharyngitis, mild to moderate. Note redness and vascularity of the pillars and uvula.

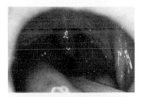

Pharyngitis, diffuse. Note redness is diffuse and intense. Cause may be viral or, if patient has fever, bacterial. If patient has no fever, exudate, or cervical lymphadenopathy, viral infection is more likely.

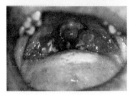

Exudative pharyngitis. A sore red throat with patches of white exudate on the tonsils is associated with streptococcal pharyngitis and some viral illnesses.

TABLE 5-11 ■ Abnormalities of the Thyroid Gland

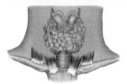

Diffuse enlargement. May result from Graves' disease, Hashimoto's thyroiditis, endemic goiter (iodine deficiency), or sporadic goiter

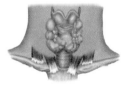

Multinodular goiter. An enlargement with two or more identifiable nodules, usually metabolic in cause

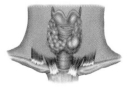

Single nodule. May result from a cyst, a benign tumor, or cancer of the thyroid, or may be one palpable nodule in a clinically unrecognized multinodular goiter

CHAPTER

The Thorax and Lungs 6

THE HEALTH HISTORY

Common or Concerning Symptoms

- Chest pain (see Table 6-1, Chest Pain, pp. 112–113)
- Dyspnea (see Table 6-2, Dyspnea, pp. 113–114)
- Wheezing
- Cough
- Blood-streaked sputum (hemoptysis)

Complaints of *chest pain* or *chest discomfort* raise the specter
of heart disease but often arise from conditions in the thorax
and lungs. For this important symptom, keep the possible
causes below in mind:

- The myocardium   Angina pectoris, myocardial
                            infarction

- The pericardium   Pericarditis

- The aorta   Dissecting aortic aneurysm

- The trachea and large   Bronchitis
  bronchi

- The parietal pleura   Pericarditis, pneumonia

■ The chest wall, including the musculoskeletal system and skin	Costochondritis, herpes zoster
■ The esophagus	Reflux esophagitis, esophageal spasm
■ Extrathoracic structures such as the neck, gallbladder, stomach	Cervical arthritis, biliary colic, gastritis

Be prepared to elicit *pulmonary complaints,* such as dyspnea, wheezing, cough, and hemoptysis.

HEALTH PROMOTION AND COUNSELING

Despite declines in smoking over the past several decades, more than 27% of Americans age 12 and older still smoke.* Regularly counsel all adults, pregnant women, parents, and adolescents who smoke to stop. Include the four **"As"**:

■ **A**sk about smoking at each visit.

■ **A**dvise patients regularly in a clear personalized message to stop smoking.

■ **A**ssist patients to set stop dates and provide educational materials for self-help.

■ **A**rrange for follow-up visits to monitor and support progress.

---

*Substance Abuse and Mental Health Services Administration, 1999 National Household Survey. www.samhsa.gov/hhsurvey/content/1999. Accessed 8/13/01.

TECHNIQUES OF EXAMINATION

SURVEY

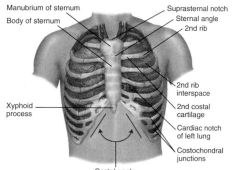

Manubrium of sternum
Body of sternum
Suprasternal notch
Sternal angle
2nd rib
2nd rib interspace
2nd costal cartilage
Cardiac notch of left lung
Costochondral junctions
Xyphoid process
Costal angle

Inspect the thorax and its respiratory movements.
Note

Techniques	Possible Findings
■ Rate, rhythm, depth, and effort of breathing	Tachypnea, hyperpnea, Cheyne–Stokes breathing
■ Inspiratory retraction of the supraclavicular areas	Occurs in chronic obstructive pulmonary disease (COPD), asthma, upper airway obstruction
■ Inspiratory contraction of the sternomastoids	Indicates severe breathing difficulty
Observe shape of patient's chest.	Normal or barrel chest (see Table 6-3, Deformities of the Thorax, p. 115–116)

TECHNIQUES	POSSIBLE FINDINGS

Listen to patient's breathing for

- Rate and rhythm of breathing

  14–16 breaths/minute in adults (see Chap. 3, p. 56)

- Stridor

  Stridor in upper airway obstruction from foreign body or epiglottitis

- Wheezes

  Wheezes in asthma and COPD

THE POSTERIOR CHEST

Inspect the chest for

- Deformities or asymmetry

  Kyphoscoliosis

- Abnormal inspiratory retraction of the interspaces

  Retraction in airway obstruction

- Impairment or unilateral lag in respiratory movement

  Disease of the underlying lung or pleura, phrenic nerve palsy

Palpate the chest for

- Tender areas

  Fractured ribs

- Assessment of visible abnormalities

  Masses, sinus tracts

TECHNIQUES	**POSSIBLE FINDINGS**

■ Chest expansion

Impairment, one or both sides

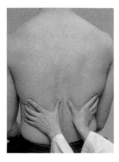

■ Tactile fremitus

Local or generalized decrease or increase

Percuss the chest in the areas illustrated, comparing one side with the other at each level, using the side-to-side "ladder pattern."

Dullness occurs when fluid or solid tissue replaces normally air-filled lung. Hyperresonance often accompanies emphysema or pneumothorax.

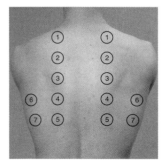

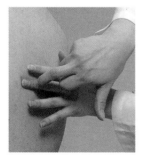

Identify level of diaphragmatic dullness on each side and **estimate** diaphragmatic excursion.

Pleural effusion or a paralyzed diaphragm raises level of dullness.

| TECHNIQUES | POSSIBLE FINDINGS |

Percussion Notes

	Relative Intensity, Pitch, and Duration	Examples
Flatness	Soft/high/short	Large pleural effusion
Dullness	Medium/medium/ medium	Lobar pneumonia
Resonance	Loud/low/long	Normal lung, simple chronic bronchitis
Hyperresonance	Louder/lower/ longer	Emphysema, pneumothorax
Tympany	Loud/high*/*	Large pneumothorax

*Distinguished mainly by musical timbre

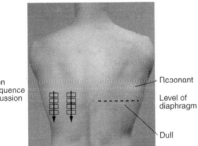

Location and sequence of percussion

Resonant

Level of diaphragm

Dull

Listen to chest with stethoscope in areas shown above, again comparing sides.	See Table 6-4, Signs in Selected Chest Disorders, p. 117.
■ Evaluate the breath sounds.	Vesicular, bronchovesicular, or bronchial breath sounds; decreased breath sounds from decreased airflow
■ Note any adventitious (added) sounds.	Crackles (fine and coarse) and continuous sounds (wheezes and rhonchi)

Breath Sounds

	Duration	Intensity and Pitch of Expiratory Sound	Example Locations
Vesicular	Insp > exp	Soft/low	Most of the lungs
Bronchovesicular	Insp = exp	Medium/ medium	1st and 2nd interspaces, interscapular area
Bronchial	Exp > insp	Loud/high	Over the manubrium; lobar pneumonia
Tracheal	Insp = exp	Very loud/ high	Over the trachea

In the figures above, duration is indicated by the length of the line, intensity by the width of the line, and pitch by the slope of the line.

Adventitious Lung Sounds

DISCONTINUOUS SOUNDS (CRACKLES OR RALES) are intermittent, nonmusical, and brief—like dots in time
  Fine crackles • • • • are soft, high pitched, and very brief (5–10 msec).
  Coarse crackles ● ● ● ● are somewhat louder, lower in pitch, and not quite so brief (20–30 msec).

CONTINUOUS SOUNDS are >250 msec, notably longer than crackles—like dashes in time—but do not necessarily persist throughout the respiratory cycle. Unlike crackles, they are musical.
  Wheezes are relatively high pitched (around 400 Hz or higher) and have a hissing or shrill quality.
  Rhonchi are relatively low pitched (around 200 Hz or lower) and have a snoring quality.

TECHNIQUES	**POSSIBLE FINDINGS**

Observe their qualities, place in the respiratory cycle, and location on the chest wall. Do they clear with deep breathing or coughing?

Assess transmitted voice sounds if you have heard bronchial breath sounds in abnormal places. Ask patient to

■ Say "99" and "ee."

Bronchophony, egophony, and whispered pectoriloquy

■ Whisper "99" or "1, 2, 3."

Transmitted Voice Sounds	
Through Normally Air-Filled Lung	**Through Airless Lung***
Spoken words muffled and indistinct	Spoken words louder, clearer (*bronchophony*)
Spoken "ee" heard as "ee"	Spoken "ee" heard as "ay" (*egophony*)
Whispered words faint and indistinct, if heard at all	Whispered words louder, clearer (*whispered pectoriloquy*)
Usually accompanied by vesicular breath sounds and normal tactile fremitus	Usually accompanied by bronchial or bronchovesicular breath sounds and increased tactile fremitus

*As in lobar pneumonia and toward the top of a large pleural effusion

While the patient is still sitting, you may inspect the breasts and examine the axillary and epitrochlear lymph nodes. Also examine the temporomandibular joint and the musculoskeletal system of the upper extremities.

TECHNIQUES	POSSIBLE FINDINGS

○— *THE ANTERIOR CHEST*

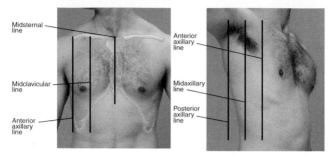

ANTERIOR VIEW   **RIGHT ANTERIOR OBLIQUE VIEW**

Inspect the chest for

■ Deformities or asymmetry	Pectus excavatum
■ Intercostal retraction	From obstructed airways
■ Impaired or lagging respiratory movement	Disease of the underlying lung or pleura, phrenic nerve palsy

Palpate the chest for

■ Tender areas	Tender pectoral muscles, costochondritis
■ Assessment of visible abnormalities	Flail chest
■ Respiratory expansion	
■ Tactile fremitus	

TECHNIQUES	POSSIBLE FINDINGS

Percuss the chest in the areas illustrated.

Normal cardiac dullness may disappear in emphysema.

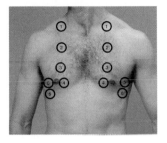

Listen to the chest with stethoscope. **Note**

■ Breath sounds

■ Adventitious sounds

■ If indicated, transmitted voice sounds

SPECIAL TECHNIQUES

ASSESSMENT OF PULMONARY FUNCTION

If appropriate, walk with patient down the hall or up a flight of stairs. Observe rate, effort, and sound of breathing, and inquire about symptoms.

FORCED EXPIRATORY TIME

Ask patient to take a deep breath in and then breathe out as quickly and completely as possible, with mouth open. Listen over trachea with

If the patient understands and cooperates well, a forced expiratory time of 6 or more seconds strongly suggests obstructive pulmonary disease.

TECHNIQUES	POSSIBLE FINDINGS

diaphragm of stethoscope, and time audible expiration. Try to get three consistent readings, allowing rests as needed.

IDENTIFICATION OF A FRACTURED RIB

Point tenderness of a rib suggests fracture but may be the result of soft-tissue injury. With one hand on the patient's sternum and the other on the thoracic spine, squeeze the patient's chest. Does this anteroposterior compression cause pain? If so, where?

Increased local rib pain, distant from your hands, suggests rib fracture rather than just soft-tissue injury.

Recording the Physical Examination– The Thorax and Lungs

"Thorax is symmetric with good expansion. Lungs resonant. Breath sounds vesicular; no rales, wheezes, or rhonchi. Diaphragms descend 4 cm bilaterally."

OR

"Thorax symmetric with moderate kyphosis and increased anteroposterior (AP) diameter, decreased expansion. Lungs are hyperresonant. Breath sounds distant with delayed expiratory phase and scattered expiratory wheezes. Fremitus decreased; no bronchophony, egophony, or whispered pectoriloquy. Diaphragms descend 2 cm bilaterally."

Suggests COPD

AIDS TO INTERPRETATION

TABLE 6-1 ■ Chest Pain

Problem and Location	Quality, Severity, and Timing	Associated Symptoms
Cardiovascular		
Angina Pectoris Retrosternal or across the anterior chest, sometimes radiating to the shoulders, arms, neck, lower jaw, or upper abdomen	**Quality:** Pressing, squeezing, tight, heavy, occasionally burning **Severity:** Mild to moderate, sometimes perceived as discomfort rather than pain **Timing:** Usually 1–3 min but up to 10 min; prolonged episodes up to 20 min	Sometimes dyspnea, nausea, swelling
Myocardial Infarction Same as in angina	**Quality:** Same as in angina **Severity:** Often but not always a severe pain **Timing:** 20 min to several hr	Nausea, vomiting, sweating, weakness
Pericarditis *Precordial:* May radiate to the tip of the shoulder and to the neck	**Quality:** Sharp, knifelike **Severity:** Often severe **Timing:** Persistent	Of the underlying illness
Retrosternal	**Quality:** Crushing **Severity:** Severe **Timing:** Persistent	Of the underlying illness

(table continues next page)

TABLE 6-1 ■ Chest Pain (Continued)

Problem and Location	Quality, Severity, and Timing	Associated Symptoms
Dissecting Aortic Aneurysm Anterior chest, radiating to the neck, back, or abdomen	**Quality:** Ripping, tearing **Severity:** Very severe **Timing:** Abrupt onset, early peak, persistent for hours or more	Syncope, hemiplegia, paraplegia
Pulmonary		
Tracheobronchitis Upper sternal or on either side of the sternum	**Quality:** Burning **Severity:** Mild to moderate **Timing:** Variable	Cough
Pleural Pain Chest wall overlying the process	**Quality:** Sharp, knifelike **Severity:** Often severe **Timing:** Persistent	Of the underlying illness
Gastrointestinal and Other		
Reflex Esophagitis Retrosternal, may radiate to the back	**Quality:** Burning, may be squeezing **Severity:** Mild to severe **Timing:** Variable	Sometimes regurgitation, dysphagia
Diffuse Esophageal Spasm Retrosternal, may radiate to the back, arms, and jaw	**Quality:** Usually squeezing **Severity:** Mild to severe **Timing:** Variable	Dysphagia
Chest Wall Pain Often below the left breast or along the costal cartilages; also elsewhere	**Quality:** Stabbing, sticking, or dull, aching **Severity:** Variable **Timing:** Fleeting to hours or days	Often local tenderness

(table continues next page)

TABLE 6-1 ■ Chest Pain *(Continued)*

Problem and Location	Quality, Severity, and Timing	Associated Symptoms
Anxiety Precordial, below the left breast, or across the anterior chest	**Quality:** Stabbing, sticking, or dull, aching **Severity:** Variable **Timing:** Fleeting to hours or days	Breathlessness, palpitations, weakness, anxiety

Note: Remember that chest pain may be referred from extrathoracic structures such as the neck (arthritis) and abdomen (biliary colic, acute cholecystitis). Pleural pain may result from abdominal conditions such as subdiaphragmatic abscess.

TABLE 6-2 ■ Dyspnea

Problem	Timing	Provoking and Relieving Factors	Associated Symptoms
Left-sided Heart Failure *(left ventricular failure or mitral stenosis)*	Dyspnea may progress slowly or suddenly, as in acute pulmonary edema	↑ by exertion, lying down ↓ by rest, sitting up, though dyspnea may become persistent	Often cough, orthopnea, paroxysmal nocturnal dyspnea, sometimes wheezing
Chronic Bronchitis*	Chronic productive cough followed by slowly progressive dyspnea	↑ by exertion, inhaled irritants, respiratory infections ↓ by expectoration, rest though dyspnea may become persistent	Chronic productive cough, recurrent respiratory infections; wheezing possible
Chronic Obstructive Pulmonary Disease (COPD)*	Slowly progressive dyspnea; relatively mild cough later	↑ by exertion ↓ by rest, though dyspnea may become persistent	Cough with scant mucoid sputum

(table continues next page)

TABLE 6-2 ■ Dyspnea *(Continued)*

Problem	Timing	Provoking and Relieving Factors	Associated Symptoms
Asthma	Acute episodes, separated by symptom-free periods; nocturnal episodes are common	↑ by allergens, irritants, respiratory infections, exercise, emotion ↓ by separation from aggravating factors	Wheezing, cough, tightness in chest
Diffuse Interstitial Lung Diseases *(sarcoidosis, widespread neoplasms, asbestosis, and idiopathic pulmonary fibrosis)*	Progressive dyspnea, which varies in its rate of development with the cause	↑ by exertion ↓ by rest, though dyspnea may become persistent	Often weakness, fatigue; cough less common than in other lung diseases
Pneumonia	An acute illness; timing varies with the causative agent		Pleuritic pain, cough, sputum, fever, though not necessarily present
Spontaneous Pneumothorax	Sudden onset of dyspnea		Pleuritic pain, cough
Acute Pulmonary Embolism	Sudden onset of dyspnea		Often none; retrosternal oppressive pain if occlusion is massive; pleuritic pain, cough, and hemoptysis may follow an embolism if pulmonary infarction ensues; symptoms of anxiety

*Chronic bronchitis and COPD may coexist.

TABLE 6-3 ■ Deformities of the Thorax

Cross Section of Thorax
Normal Adult

The thorax in the normal adult is wider than it is deep. Its lateral diameter is larger than its anteroposterior diameter.

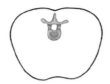

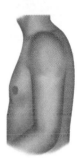

Barrel Chest

A barrel chest has an increased anteroposterior diameter. This shape is normal during infancy, and often accompanies normal aging and chronic obstructive pulmonary disease.

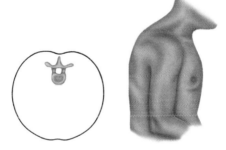

Traumatic Flail Chest

If multiple ribs are fractured, paradoxical movements of the thorax may be seen. As descent of the diaphragm decreases intrathoracic pressure on inspiration, the injured area caves inward; on expiration, it moves outward.

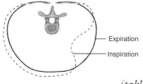

Expiration
Inspiration

(table continues next page)

TABLE 6-3 ■ Deformities of the Thorax *(Continued)*

Funnel Chest (*Pectus Excavatum*)

A funnel chest is characterized by a depression in the lower portion of the sternum. Compression of the heart and great vessels may cause murmurs.

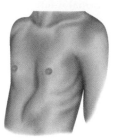

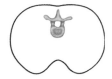

Cross Section of Thorax
Pigeon Chest (*Pectus Carinatum*)

In a pigeon chest, the sternum is displaced anteriorly, increasing the anteroposterior diameter. The costal cartilages adjacent to the protruding sternum are depressed.

Depressed costal cartilages

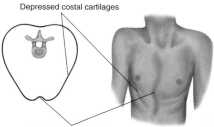

Anteriorly displaced sternum

Thoracic Kyphoscoliosis

In thoracic kyphoscoliosis, abnormal spinal curvatures and vertebral rotation deform the chest. Distortion of the underlying lungs may make interpretation of lung findings very difficult.

Spinal convexity to the right
(patient bending forward)

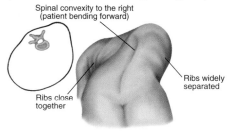

Ribs widely separated

Ribs close together

TABLE 6-4 ■ Signs in Selected Chest Disorders

	Trachea	Percussion Note	Breath Sounds	Transmitted Voice Sounds	Adventitious Sounds
Chronic Bronchitis	Midline	Resonant	Normal	Normal	None, or wheezes, rhonchi, crackles
Left Heart Failure (early)	Midline	Resonant	Normal	Normal	Late inspiratory crackles in lower lungs; possible wheezes
Consolidation*	Midline	Dull	Bronchial	Increased[†]	Late inspiratory crackles
Atelectasis (Lobar)	May be shifted *toward*	Dull	Usually absent	Usually absent	None
Pleural Effusion (large)	May be shifted *away*	Dull	Decreased to absent	Decreased to absent	Usually none, possible pleural rub
Pneumothorax	May be shifted *away*	Hyperresonant or tympanitic	Decreased to absent	Decreased to absent	Possible pleural rub
COPD	Midline	Hyperresorant	Decreased to absent	Decreased	None unless bronchitis also
Asthma	Midline	Resonant to hyperresonant	May be obscured by wheezes	Decreased	Wheezes, perhaps crackles

*As in lobar pneumonia, pulmonary edema, or pulmonary hemorrhage

[†]With increased tactile fremitus, bronchophony, egophony, whispered pectoriloquy

The Cardiovascular System

THE HEALTH HISTORY

Common or Concerning Symptoms

- Chest pain
- Palpitations
- Shortness of breath, orthopnea, or paroxysmal nocturnal dyspnea
- Swelling or edema

As you listen to complaints of *chest pain or discomfort,* keep serious adverse events in mind, such as *angina pectoris, myocardial infarction,* or even a *dissecting aortic aneurysm.* Ask also about palpitations, orthopnea, paroxysmal nocturnal dyspnea (PND), and edema.

- *Palpitations* are an unpleasant awareness of the heartbeat.

- *Shortness of breath* may be reported as dyspnea, orthopnea, or PND.

- *Dyspnea* is an uncomfortable awareness of breathing that is inappropriate to a given level of exertion.

- *Orthopnea* is dyspnea that occurs when the patient is lying down and improves when the patient sits up. It suggests *left ventricular heart failure* or *mitral stenosis;* it also may accompany *obstructive lung disease.*

- *PND* describes episodes of sudden dyspnea and orthopnea that awaken the patient from sleep, usually 1 to 2 hours after going to bed, prompting the patient to sit up, stand up, or go to a window for air.

- *Edema* refers to the accumulation of excessive fluid in the interstitial tissue spaces; it appears as swelling. *Dependent edema* appears in the lowest body parts (feet and lower legs) when sitting or in the sacrum when bedridden.

HEALTH PROMOTION AND COUNSELING

Important Topics for Health Promotion and Counseling

- Cholesterol level
- Lifestyle management: diet, weight reduction, exercise, smoking
- Screening for hypertension

In May 2001, the National Heart, Lung, and Blood Institute of the National Institutes of Health published the *Third Report of the National Cholesterol Education Program Expert Panel,* which sets standards for the detection, evaluation, and treatment of high cholesterol levels in adults.*

Your advice about risk reduction should cover lifestyle changes, including diet, weight reduction, and exercise, as well as drug therapy when indicated. For counseling about weight, apply the principles for assessing *body mass index* enumerated in Chapter 3 (pp. 35–36 and 50–51).

---

*Third Report of the National Cholesterol Education Program (NCEP) Expert Panel. Detection, Evaluation, and Treatment of High Blood Cholesterol in Adults–Executive Summary. National Cholesterol Education Program, National Heart, Lung, and Blood Institute, National Institutes of Health. NIH Publication No. 01-3670. May 2001. www.nhlbi.nih.gov/guidelines/cholesterol/index.htm. Accessed 10/8/02.

STANDARDS FOR DETECTION AND EVALUATION OF CHOLESTEROL

- *Obtain a fasting lipid profile* in all adults 20 years of age or older once every 5 years. Targets for optimal lipid levels (mg/dL) are as follows:
  - LDL cholesterol   <100
  - Total cholesterol   <200
  - HDL cholesterol   <40 is low; ≥60 is high
- *Assess additional major risk factors and "risk equivalents."* Risk *factors* are smoking, hypertension if blood pressure is greater than 140/90 mm Hg or the patient is using medication, HDL less than 40 mg/dL, family history of premature coronary heart disease (CHD) (affected male first-degree relative younger than 55 years; affected female first-degree relative younger than 65 years), and age, namely men 45 years of age or older and women 55 years of age or older. *Risk equivalents* include diabetes; other forms of atherosclerotic disease—peripheral vascular disease, abdominal aortic aneurysm, and symptomatic carotid artery disease; and two or more risk factors, raising the 10-year risk of CHD to more than 20%.
- The desired goal for the patient's LDL level varies according to the number of risk factors.

Risk Category	LDL Level Goal (mg/dL)
0–1 risk factor	<160
2+ or multiple risk factors	<130
CHD or CHD risk equivalents	<100

- Additional treatment is recommended if the triglyceride level exceeds 200 mg/dL.

TECHNIQUES OF EXAMINATION

HEART RATE AND BLOOD PRESSURE

If not already done, measure the radial or apical pulse. **Estimate** systolic blood pressure by palpation and **add** 30 mm Hg. Use this sum as the target for further cuff inflations.

This step helps you to detect an auscultatory gap.

Measure blood pressure with a sphygmomanometer. If indicated, **check** it.

Orthostatic (postural) hypotension (with position change of supine to sitting, or sitting to standing, BP↓ ≥10 mm Hg; HR↑ ≥20 beats/min)

JUGULAR VEINS

Identify *jugular venous pulsations* and their highest point in the neck. Adjust angle of the bed as necessary.

Measure *jugular venous pressure* (JVP)—the vertical distance between this highest point and the sternal angle, normally less than 3–4 cm.

Elevated JVP in right-sided heart failure; decreased JVP in hypovolemia from dehydration or gastrointestinal bleeding

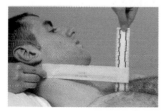

TECHNIQUES	POSSIBLE FINDINGS
Study the venous pulse waves. Note the *a* wave of atrial contraction and the *v* wave of venous filling.	Absent *a* waves in atrial fibrillation; prominent *v* waves in tricuspid regurgitation.

CAROTID PULSE

Assess the amplitude and contour of the carotid upstroke.	A *delayed* upstroke in carotid stenosis; a *bounding* upstroke in aortic insufficiency
Listen for bruits.	Carotid bruits suggest atherosclerotic narrowing.

THE HEART

Sequence of the Cardiac Examination

Patient Position	Examination
Supine, with the head elevated 30°	Inspect and palpate the precordium: the 2nd interspaces; the right ventricle; and the left ventricle, including the apical impulse (diameter, location, amplitude, duration).
Left lateral decubitus	Palpate the apical impulse if not previously detected. Listen at the apex with the bell of the stethoscope for low-pitched extra sounds (S_3, opening snap, diastolic rumble of mitral stenosis).
Supine, with the head elevated 30°	Listen at the tricuspid area with the bell. Listen at all the auscultatory areas with the diaphragm.
Sitting, leaning forward, after full exhalation	Listen along the left sternal border and at the apex for the soft decrescendo diastolic murmur of aortic insufficiency.

TECHNIQUES	**POSSIBLE FINDINGS**

Inspect and **palpate** the anterior chest for pulsations.

Identify the *apical impulse*. Turn patient to left as necessary. **Note**

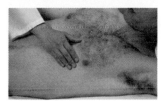

- Location of impulse

  Displaced to left in pregnancy

- Diameter

  Increased diameter, amplitude, and duration in left ventricular dilatation, as in congestive heart failure (CHF)

- Amplitude—usually *tapping*

  Sustained in left ventricular hypertrophy; *diffuse* in CHF

- Duration

Feel for a right ventricular impulse in left parasternal and epigastric areas.

Prominent impulses suggest right ventricular enlargement.

Palpate left and right second interspaces close to sternum. **Note** any thrills in these areas.

Pulsations of great vessels; accentuated S_2; thrills of aortic or pulmonic stenosis

Listen to heart with stethoscope in the areas illustrated.

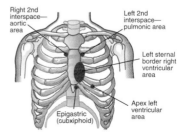

Right 2nd interspace— aortic area

Left 2nd interspace— pulmonic area

Left sternal border right ventricular area

Apex left ventricular area

Epigastric (cubxiphoid)

TECHNIQUES	POSSIBLE FINDINGS
Use the *diaphragm* in the areas illustrated above for relatively *high-pitched sounds* like S_1, S_2.	Also murmurs of aortic and mitral regurgitation; pericardial friction rubs
Use the *bell* for *low-pitched sounds* at the lower left sternal border and apex.	S_3, S_4, murmur of mitral stenosis
Listen at each area for:	See Table 7-1, Heart Sounds, p. 129; Table 7-2, Variations in the First Heart Sound (S_1), p. 130; Table 7-3, Variations in the Second Heart Sound (S_2), pp. 131–132.
■ S_1	
■ S_2. Is splitting normal in left 2nd and 3rd interspaces?	Physiologic (inspiratory) or pathologic (expiratory) splitting
■ Extra sounds in systole	Systolic clicks
■ Extra sounds in diastole	S_3, S_4
■ Systolic murmurs	Midsystolic, pansystolic, late systolic murmurs
■ Diastolic murmurs	Early, mid-, or late diastolic murmurs
Identify, if murmurs are present, their	
■ Timing in the cardiac cycle (systole, diastole)	See Table 7-4, Heart Murmurs and Similar Sounds, pp. 133–134.
■ Shape	Plateau, crescendo, decrescendo

TECHNIQUES	POSSIBLE FINDINGS
	A *crescendo–decrescendo murmur* first rises in intensity, then falls.
	A *plateau murmur* has the same intensity throughout.
	A *crescendo murmur* grows louder.
	A *decrescendo murmur* grows softer.

- Location of maximal intensity

- Radiation

- Intensity on a 6-point scale

See "Gradations of Murmurs"

- Pitch

High, medium, low

- Quality

Blowing, harsh, musical, rumbling

Listen at the apex with patient turned toward left side.

Left-sided S_3, S_4, and diastolic murmur of mitral stenosis

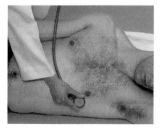

Gradations of Murmurs

Grade	Description
Grade 1	Very faint, heard only after listener has "tuned in"; may not be heard in all positions
Grade 2	Quiet, but heard immediately after placing the stethoscope on the chest
Grade 3	Moderately loud
Grade 4	Loud, with palpable thrill
Grade 5	Very loud, with thrill. May be heard when the stethoscope is partly off the chest
Grade 6	Very loud, with thrill. May be heard with stethoscope entirely off the chest

Listen down left sternal border to the apex as patient sits, leaning forward, with breath held in exhalation.

Diastolic decrescendo murmur of aortic regurgitation

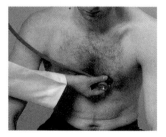

TECHNIQUES	POSSIBLE FINDINGS

SPECIAL TECHNIQUES

∿ / ⌐ PULSUS ALTERANS

Feel pulse for alternation in amplitude. Lower pressure of blood pressure cuff slowly to systolic level while you listen with stethoscope over brachial artery.

Alternating amplitude of pulse or sudden doubling of Korotkoff sounds indicate pulsus alterans—a sign of left ventricular failure.

PARADOXICAL PULSE

Lower pressure of blood pressure cuff slowly and note two pressure levels: (1) where Korotkoff sounds are first heard, and (2) where they first persist through the respiratory cycle. These levels are normally not more than 3–4 mm Hg apart.

A drop of greater than 10 mm Hg during inspiration signifies a paradoxical pulse. Consider obstructive lung disease, pericardial tamponade, or constrictive pericarditis.

∿ VALSALVA MANEUVER

Ask patient to strain down. In suspected *mitral valve prolapse (MVP)*, listen to the timing of click and murmur.

Ventricular filling decreases, the systolic click of MVP is earlier, and the murmur lengthens.

To distinguish *aortic stenosis (AS)* from *hypertrophic cardiomyopathy (HC)*, listen to the intensity of the murmur.

In AS, the murmur decreases; in HC, it often increases.

⌐/⌐ SQUATTING AND STANDING

In suspected *MVP*, listen for the click and murmur in both positions.

Squatting increases ventricular filling and delays the click and murmur. Standing reverses the changes.

TECHNIQUES	**POSSIBLE FINDINGS**
Try to distinguish *AS* from *HC* by listening to the murmur in both positions.	Squatting increases murmur of AS and decreases murmur of HC. Standing reverses the changes.

Recording the Physical Examination—The Cardiovascular Examination

"The jugular venous pulse (JVP) is 3 cm above the sternal angle with the head of the bed elevated to 30°. Carotid upstrokes are brisk, without bruits. The point of maximal impulse (PMI) is tapping, 7 cm lateral to the midsternal line in the 5th intercostal space. Good S_1 and S_2. No murmurs or extra sounds."

OR

"The JVP is 5 cm above the sternal angle with the head of bed elevated to 50°. Carotid upstrokes are brisk; a bruit is heard over the left carotid artery. The PMI is diffuse, 3 cm in diameter, palpated at the anterior axillary line in the 5th and 6th intercostal spaces. S_1 and S_2 are soft. S_3 present. Harsh 2/6 holosystolic murmur best heard at the apex, radiating to the lower left sternal border (LLSB). No S_4 or diastolic murmurs."

Suggests CHF with possible left carotid occlusion and mitral regurgitation

AIDS TO INTERPRETATION

TABLE 7-1 ■ Heart Sounds

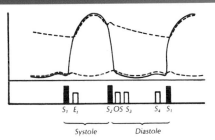

Finding	Possible Causes
S_1 accentuated	Tachycardia, states of high cardiac output; mitral stenosis
S_1 diminished	First-degree heart block; reduced left ventricular contractility; immobile mitral valve, as in mitral regurgitation
Systolic clicks(s)	Mitral valve prolapse
S_2 accentuated in right 2nd interspace	Systemic hypertension, dilated aortic root
S_2 diminished or absent in right 2nd Interspace	Immobile aortic valve, as in calcific aortic stenosis
P_2 accentuated	Pulmonary hypertension, dilated pulmonary artery, atrial septal defect
P_2 diminished or absent	Aging, pulmonic stenosis
Opening snap	Mitral stenosis
S_3	Physiologic (usually in children and young adults); pathologic myocardial failure, volume overload of a ventricle, as in mitral regurgitation
S_4	Excellent physical conditioning (trained athletes); resistance to ventricular filling because of decreased compliance, as in hypertensive heart disease or left ventricular hypertrophy

TABLE 7-2 ■ Variations in the First Heart Sound (S₁)

Normal Variations

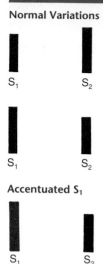

S_1 is softer than S_2 at the **base** (right and left 2nd interspaces).

S_1 is often but not always louder than S_2 at the **apex.**

Accentuated S₁

S_1 occurs in (1) tachycardia, rhythms with a short PR interval, and high cardiac output states (e.g., exercise, anemia, hyperthyroidism), and (2) mitral stenosis.

Diminished S₁

This occurs in first-degree heart block, calcified mitral valve of mitral regurgitation, and left ventricular contractility of congestive heart failure or coronary heart disease.

Varying S₁

S_1 varies in complete heart block, and any totally irregular rhythm (e.g., atrial fibrillation).

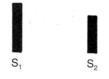

Split S₁

This is normally along the **lower left sternal border** if audible tricuspid component; also at **apex** if an S_4, an aortic ejection sound, an early systolic click, right bundle branch block, and premature ventricular contractions.

TABLE 7-3 ■ Variations in the Second Heart Sound (S₂)

Expiration	Inspiration

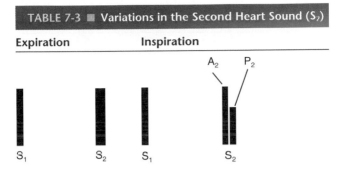

Physiologic Splitting of S₂ in the 2nd or 3rd left interspace. The pulmonic component of S₂ is usually too faint to be heard at the apex or aortic area, where S₂ is single and derived from aortic valve closure alone. Accentuated by inspiration; usually disappears on exertion.

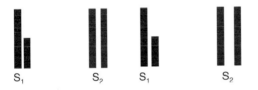

Pathologic Splitting. Wide splitting of S₂ persists throughout the respiratory cycle; from delayed closure of the pulmonic valve (e.g., by pulmonic stenosis or right bundle branch block), also from early closure of the aortic valve, as in mitral regurgitation.

Fixed Splitting does not vary with respiration, as in atrial septal defect, right ventricular failure.

(table continues next page)

TABLE 7-3 ■ Variations in the Second Heart Sound (S_2) (Continued)

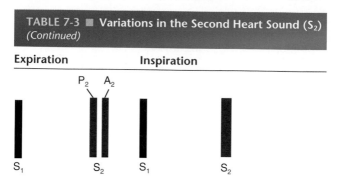

Paradoxical or Reversed Splitting appears on expiration and disappears on inspiration. Closure of the aortic valve is abnormally delayed, so A_2 follows P_2 on expiration, as in left bundle branch block.

More on A_2 and P_2

Increased Intensity of A_2, Second Right Interspace (where only A_2 can usually be heard) occurs in systemic hypertension because of the increased pressure. It also occurs when the aortic root is dilated, probably because the aortic valve is then closer to the chest wall.

Decreased or Absent A_2, Second Right Interspace is noted in calcific aortic stenosis because of immobility of the valve. If A_2 is inaudible, no splitting is heard.

Increased Intensity of P_2. When P_2 is equal to or louder than A_2, pulmonary hypertension may be suspected. Other causes include a dilated pulmonary artery and an atrial septal defect. Splitting of the second heart sound that is heard widely, even at the apex and the right base, indicates an accentuated P_2.

Decreased or Absent P_2 is most commonly due to the increased anteroposterior diameter of the chest associated with aging. It can also result from pulmonic stenosis. If P_2 is inaudible, no splitting is heard.

TABLE 7-4 ■ Heart Murmurs and Similar Sounds

	Likely Causes
Midsystolic	Innocent murmurs (no cardiovascular abnormality)
	Physiologic murmurs (from increased flow across a semilunar valve, as in pregnancy, fever, anemia)
	Aortic stenosis
	Murmurs that mimic aortic stenosis (aortic sclerosis, bicuspid aortic valve, dilated aorta, and pathologically increased systolic flow across the aortic valve)
	Hypertrophic cardiomyopathy
	Pulmonic stenosis
Pansystolic	Mitral regurgitation
	Tricuspid regurgitation
	Ventricular septal defect
Late Systolic	Mitral valve prolapse
Early Diastolic	Aortic regurgitation
Middiastolic and Presystolic	Mitral stenosis

(table continues next page)

TABLE 7-4 ■ Heart Murmurs and Similar Sounds
(Continued)

Likely Causes

Continuous Murmurs and Murmurlike Sounds

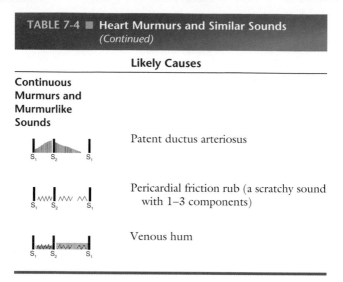

Patent ductus arteriosus

Pericardial friction rub (a scratchy sound with 1–3 components)

Venous hum

The Breasts and Axillae

Common or Concerning Symptoms

- Breast lump or mass
- Breast pain or discomfort
- Nipple discharge

Ask, "Do you examine your breasts?" . . . "How often?" Ask about any *lumps, pain,* or *discomfort* in the breasts. Also ask about any *discharge from the nipples.*

HEALTH PROMOTION AND COUNSELING

Important Topics for Health Promotion and Counseling

- Risk factors for breast cancer
- Breast cancer screening
- Breast self-examination (BSE)

Breast masses show marked variation in etiology, from fibroadenomas and cysts seen in younger women, to abscess or mastitis, to primary breast cancer. All breast masses warrant careful evaluation, and definitive diagnostic measures should be pursued.

Palpable Masses of the Breast		
Age	Common Lesion	Characteristics
15–25	Fibroadenoma	Usually fine, round, mobile, nontender
25–50	Cysts	Usually soft to firm, round, mobile; often tender
	Fibrocystic changes	Nodular, ropelike
	Cancer	Irregular, stellate, firm, not clearly delineated from surrounding tissue
50 or older	Cancer until proven otherwise	As above
Pregnancy/ lactation	Lactating adenomas, cysts, mastitis, and cancer	As above

(Adapted from Schultz MZ, Ward BA, Reiss M: Ch. 149. Breast Diseases. In Noble J, Greene HL, Levinson W, Modest GA, Young MJ (eds): Primary Care Medicine, 2nd ed. St. Louis, Mosby, 1996.)

Risk Factors for Breast Cancer. Although 70% of affected women have no known predisposing factors, definite risk factors are well established. You may wish to use the Breast Cancer Risk Assessment Tool of the National Cancer Institute (www.brca.nci.gov) or other available clinical models, such as the Gail model.

Breast Cancer Screening. Teaching all women the *breast self-examination* (BSE) promotes health awareness. The American Cancer Society recommends:

■ Monthly BSE beginning at 20 years of age

■ *Clinical breast examination* (CBE) by a health care professional every 3 years for women between 20 and 39 years of age, and annually after 40 years of age

■ Yearly *mammography* for women 40 years of age and older.* For women at increased risk, many clinicians advise a screening mammography at 35 or 40 years of age, then every 2 to 3 years until 50 years of age.

Summary of Breast Cancer Risk Factors

Factor	Relative Risk (%)
Family History	
First-degree relative with breast cancer	1.2–3.0
Premenopausal	3.1
Premenopausal and bilateral	8.5–9.0
Postmenopausal	1.5
Postmenopausal and bilateral	4.0–5.4
Menstrual History	
Age at menarche <12 years	1.3
Age at menopause >55 years	1.5–2.0
Pregnancy	
First live birth from 25–29 years	1.5
First live birth after 30 years	1.9
First live birth after 35 years	2.0–3.0
Nulliparous	3.0
Breast Conditions and Diseases	
Nonproliferative disease	1.0
Proliferative disease	1.9
Proliferative with atypical hyperplasia	4.4
Lobular carcinoma in situ	6.9–12.0

(Adapted from Bilmoria MM and Morrow M: The woman at increased risk for breast cancer: evaluation and management strategies. Ca 45(5):263, 1995. See also American Cancer Society, www.cancer.org.)

*American Cancer Society. www.cancer.org. Accessed 9/23/02.

TECHNIQUES	POSSIBLE FINDINGS

TECHNIQUES OF EXAMINATION

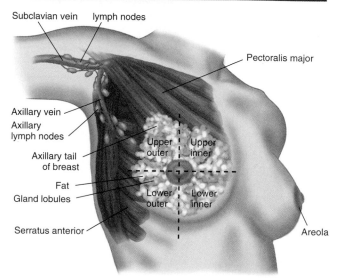

THE FEMALE BREAST

Inspect the breasts in four positions for

■ Size and symmetry	Development, asymmetry
■ Contour	Flattening, dimpling
■ Appearance of the skin	Edema (peau d'orange) in breast cancer

TECHNIQUES	POSSIBLE FINDINGS

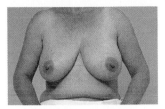

ARMS AT SIDES

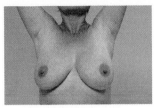

ARMS OVER HEAD

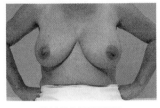

HANDS PRESSED AGAINST HIPS

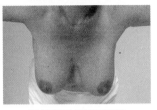

LEANING FORWARD

Inspect the nipples.

- Compare their size, shape, and direction of pointing.

  Inversion, retraction, deviation

- Note any rashes, ulcerations, or discharge.

  Paget's disease of the nipple, galactorrhea

○ **Palpate** the breasts for

- Consistency

  Physiologic nodularity

- Tenderness

  Infection, premenstrual tenderness

- Nodules. If present, **note** *location, size, shape, consistency, delimitation, tenderness,* and *mobility.*

  Cyst, fibroadenoma, cancer

Palpation is best performed when the breast tissue is

TECHNIQUES	**POSSIBLE FINDINGS**

flattened and the patient is supine. Palpate a rectangular area extending from the clavicle to the inframammary fold or bra line, and from the midsternal line to the posterior axillary line and well into the axilla for the tail of Spence.

Use *vertical strip pattern* (currently the best validated technique for detecting breast masses) or a circular or wedge pattern. Palpate in *small, concentric circles.*

■ For *the lateral portion of the breast*, ask the patient to roll onto the opposite hip, placing her hand on her forehead but keeping shoulders pressed against the bed or examining table.

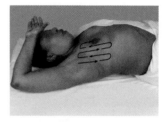

■ For *the medial portion of the breast*, ask the patient to lie with her shoulders flat against the bed or examining table, placing her hand at her neck and lifting up her elbow until it is even with her shoulder.

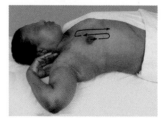

Palpate each nipple.   Thickening in cancer

TECHNIQUES	**POSSIBLE FINDINGS**

THE MALE BREAST

Inspect the nipple and areola.	Gynecomastia, cancer
Palpate the areola and adjacent area.	Gynecomastia, cancer, fat

AXILLAE

Inspect for rashes, infection, and pigmentation.	Hidradenitis suppurativa, acanthosis nigricans
Palpate the central axillary nodes.	Lymphadenopathy

If indicated, **palpate** the other axillary nodes:

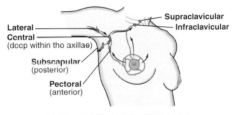

Lateral
Central
(deep within the axillae)
Subscapular
(posterior)
Pectoral
(anterior)
Supraclavicular
Infraclavicular

ARROWS INDICATE DIRECTION OF LYMPH FLOW

- Pectoral group

- Lateral group

- Subscapular group

TECHNIQUES	POSSIBLE FINDINGS

SPECIAL TECHNIQUE

○— **BREAST DISCHARGE**

Compress the areola in a spokelike pattern around the nipple if patient has reported spontaneous nipple discharge. **Watch** for discharge.

Type and source of discharge may thereby be identified.

PATIENT INSTRUCTIONS FOR THE BREAST SELF-EXAMINATION (BSE)

Lying Supine

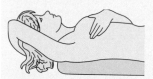
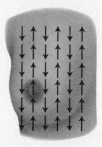

1. Lie down with a pillow under your right shoulder. Place your right arm behind your head.
2. Use the finger pads of the three middle fingers on your left hand to feel for lumps in the right breast. The finger pads are the top third of each finger.
3. Press firmly enough to know how your breast feels. A firm ridge in the lower curve of each breast is normal. If you're not sure how hard to press, talk with your health care provider, or try to copy the way the doctor or nurse does it.
4. Press firmly on the breast in an up-and-down or "strip" pattern. You can also use a circular or wedge pattern, but be
(continued)

sure to use the same pattern every time. Check the entire breast area, and remember how your breast feels from month to month.

5. Repeat the examination on your left breast, using the finger pads of the right hand.
6. If you find any changes, see your doctor right away.

Standing

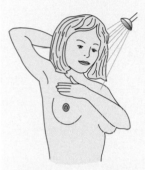

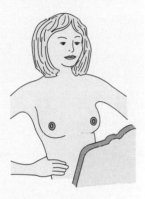

1. Repeat the examination of both breasts while standing, with one arm behind your head. The upright position makes it easier to check the upper outer part of the breasts (toward your armpit). This is where about half of breast cancers are found. You may want to do the upright part of the BSE while you are in the shower. Your soapy hands will make it easy to check how your breasts feel as they glide over the wet skin.

2. For added safety, you might want to check your breasts by standing in front of a mirror right after your BSE each month. See if there are any changes in the way your breasts look, such as dimpling of the skin, changes in the nipple, redness, or swelling.

3. If you find any changes, see your doctor right away.

(Adapted from the American Cancer Society, www.cancer.org. Accessed 9/1/01.)

Recording the Physical Examination— Breasts and Axillae

"Breasts symmetric and without masses. Nipples without discharge." (Axillary adenopathy usually included after Neck in section on Lymph Nodes, see p. 82.)

OR

"Breasts pendulous with diffuse fibrocystic changes. Single firm 1 × 1 cm mass, mobile and nontender, with overlying peau d'orange appearance in right breast, upper outer quadrant at 11 o'clock."

Suggests possible breast cancer

AIDS TO INTERPRETATION

TABLE 8-1 ■ Visible Signs of Breast Cancer

Retraction Signs

Mechanism

As breast cancer advances, it causes fibrosis, producing retraction signs: dimpling, changes in contour, and retraction or deviation of the nipple. Other causes of retraction include fat necrosis and mammary duct ectasia.

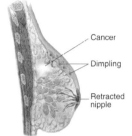

Skin Dimpling

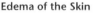

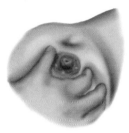

Edema of the Skin

From lymphatic blockade, appearing as thickened skin with enlarged pores—the so-called *peau d'orange* (orange peel) *sign.*

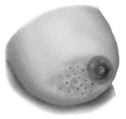

(table continues next page)

TABLE 8-1 ■ Visible Signs of Breast Cancer *(Continued)*

Abnormal Contours
Look for any variation in the normal convexity of each breast, and compare one side with the other.

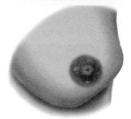

Nipple Retraction and Deviation
A retracted nipple is flattened or pulled inward. It may also be broadened and feel thickened. The nipple may deviate, or point in a different direction, typically toward the underlying cancer.

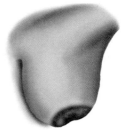

Paget's Disease of the Nipple
An uncommon form of breast cancer that usually starts as a scaly, eczemalike lesion. The skin may also weep, crust, or erode. A breast mass may be present. Suspect Paget's disease in any persisting dermatitis of the nipple and areola.

Dermatitis of areola

Erosion of nipple

The Abdomen

THE HEALTH HISTORY

Common or Concerning Symptoms

Gastrointestinal Disorders

- Indigestion or anorexia
- Nausea, vomiting, or hematemesis
- Abdominal pain
- Dysphagia and/ or odynophagia
- Change in bowel function
- Constipation or diarrhea
- Jaundice

Urinary and Renal Disorders

- Suprapubic pain
- Dysuria, urgency, or frequency
- Hesitancy, decreased stream in males
- Polyuria or nocturia
- Urinary incontinence
- Hematuria
- Kidney or flank pain
- Ureteral colic

THE GASTROINTESTINAL TRACT

Patients often complain of *indigestion*. Find out just what your patient means. Possibilities include:

- *Heartburn*

Suggests gastric acid reflux

- *Excessive gas,* especially with frequent belching, abdominal bloating or distention, or *flatus,* the passage of gas by rectum, normally about 600 ml per day

- Unpleasant *abdominal fullness* after normal meals or *early satiety,* the inability to eat a full meal

Consider diabetic gastroparesis, anticholinergic drugs, gastric outlet obstruction, and gastric cancer. Early satiety may signify hepatitis.

- *Nausea and vomiting*

- *Abdominal pain*

Abdominal pain warrants careful clinical assessment. Be familiar with three broad categories:

- *Visceral pain* occurs when hollow abdominal organs such as the intestine or biliary tree contract unusually forcefully or are distended or stretched. It may be difficult to localize. It varies in quality and may be gnawing, burning, cramping, or aching. When severe, it may be associated with sweating, pallor, nausea, vomiting, and restlessness.

Visceral pain in the right upper quadrant (RUQ) from liver distention against its capsule in alcoholic hepatitis

- *Parietal pain,* from inflammation of the parietal peritoneum, is steady, aching, and usually more severe and more precisely localized over the involved structure than is visceral pain.

Visceral periumbilical pain in early acute appendicitis from distention of inflamed appendix gradually changes to parietal pain in the right lower quadrant (RLQ) from inflammation of the adjacent parietal peritoneum.

- *Referred pain* occurs in more distant sites that are innervated at approximately the same spinal levels as the disordered structure.

Pain of duodenal or pancreatic origin may be referred to the back. Pain from the biliary tree may be referred to the right shoulder or right posterior chest.

- Pain from the chest, spine, or pelvis may be referred to the abdomen.

Pain from pleurisy or acute myocardial infarction may be referred to the upper abdomen.

Ask patients to *describe the abdominal pain in their own words,* then ask them to *point to the pain.* Pursue important details: "Where does the pain start?" "Does it radiate or travel?" "What is the pain like?" "How severe is it?" "How about on a scale of 1 to 10?" "What makes it better or worse?"

Elicit any *symptoms associated with the pain,* such as fever or chills, and ask their sequence.

In some patients, you will be struck by *jaundice* or *icterus,* the yellowish discoloration of the skin and sclerae from increased levels of bilirubin, a bile pigment derived chiefly from the breakdown of hemoglobin. *Intrahepatic jaundice* can be *hepatocellular,* from damage to the hepatocytes, or *cholestatic,* from impaired excretion caused by damaged hepatocytes or intrahepatic bile ducts. *Extrahepatic jaundice* arises from obstructed extrahepatic bile ducts, most commonly the cystic and common bile ducts.

Obstruction of the common bile duct by gallstones or pancreatic carcinoma

Ask about associated symptoms. What was the *color of the urine* as the patient became ill? Increased levels of conjugated bilirubin in the blood may be excreted into the urine, turning the urine a dark yellowish brown or tea color.

Dark urine from bilirubin indicates impaired excretion of bilirubin into the gastrointestinal tract.

Ask also about the *color of the stools.* When excretion of bile into the intestine is obstructed completely, stools become gray or light-colored, or *acholic,* without bile.

Acholic stools briefly in viral hepatitis, common in obstructive jaundice

RISK FACTORS FOR LIVER DISEASE

- *Hepatitis:* Travel or meals in areas with poor sanitation, ingestion of contaminated water or foodstuffs (hepatitis A); parenteral or mucous membrane exposure to infectious body fluids such as blood, serum, semen, and saliva, especially through sexual contact with an infected partner or use of shared needles for injection drug use (hepatitis B); illicit intravenous drug use or blood transfusion (hepatitis C)
- *Alcoholic hepatitis* or *alcoholic cirrhosis:* interview the patient carefully about alcohol use
- *Toxic liver damage* from medications, industrial solvents, or environmental toxins
- *Extrahepatic biliary obstruction:* resulting from gallbladder disease or surgery
- *Hereditary disorders* in the Family History

THE URINARY TRACT

With infection or irritation of either the bladder or urethra, ask about *pain on urination,* usually felt as a burning sensation. Some clinicians refer to this as *dysuria,* while others reserve the term dysuria for difficulty voiding. Women may report internal urethral discomfort, sometimes described as a pressure, or external burning from the flow of urine across irritated or inflamed labia. Men typically feel a burning sensation proximal to the glans penis. In contrast, *prostatic pain* occurs in the perineum and occasionally in the rectum.

Also consider bladder stones, foreign bodies, tumors, and acute prostatitis. In women, internal burning in urethritis, external burning in vulvovaginitis

Other associated symptoms include urinary *urgency,* an unusually intense and immediate desire to void, sometimes leading to involuntary voiding or *urge incontinence;* urinary *frequency,* or abnormally frequent voiding; fever or chills; blood in the urine; or any pain in the abdomen, flank, or back.

Men with partially obstructed urinary outflow often report *hesitancy* in starting the urine stream, *straining to void, reduced caliber and force of the urine stream,* or *dribbling* as they complete voiding.

Be sure to assess for any *polyuria,* a significant increase in 24-hour urine volume; *nocturia,* urinary frequency at night; or *urinary incontinence,* involuntary loss of urine that may become socially embarrassing or cause problems with hygiene.

See Table 9-2, Urinary Incontinence, pp. 167–168.

Find out if the patient leaks small amounts of urine with coughing, sneezing, laughing, or lifting. Is it difficult for the patient to hold the urine once there is an urge to void, with loss of large amounts of urine? Is there a sensation of bladder fullness and frequent leaking

Stress incontinence with increased intra-abdominal pressure from decreased contractility of urethral sphincter or poor support of bladder neck; *urge incontinence* if unable to hold the urine, from detrusor overactivity; *overflow incontinence* when

or voiding of small amounts, but difficulty emptying the bladder?

the bladder cannot be emptied until bladder pressure exceeds urethral pressure, from anatomic obstruction by prostatic hypertrophy or stricture, also neurogenic abnormalities

In addition, the patient's functional status may affect voiding behaviors significantly.

Functional incontinence from impaired cognition, musculoskeletal problems, immobility

Patients also may complain of *kidney pain,* often reported as *flank pain,* and typically dull, aching, and steady.

Kidney pain occurs in acute pyelonephritis.

Ureteral pain is usually severe and colicky.

Sudden obstruction of a ureter, as by urinary stones or blood clots, causes renal or ureteral colic.

HEALTH PROMOTION AND COUNSELING

Important Topics for Health Promotion and Counseling

- Screening for alcohol and substance abuse
- Risk factors for hepatitis A, B, and C
- Screening for colon cancer

Assessing *use of alcohol and other substances* is a primary responsibility. Focus on detection, counseling, and, for significant impairment, specific treatment recommendations.

Use the four CAGE questions to screen for alcohol dependence or abuse in all adolescents and adults, including pregnant women (see Chap. 2). Brief counseling interventions have been shown to reduce alcohol consumption by up to 25%.*

Protective measures against *infectious hepatitis* include counseling about transmission:

■ *Hepatitis A:* Transmission is fecal–oral. Illness occurs approximately 30 days after exposure. Hepatitis A vaccine is recommended for travelers to endemic areas; food handlers; military personnel; caretakers of children; Native Americans and Alaska Natives; selected health care, sanitation, and laboratory workers; homosexual men; and injection drug users.

■ *Hepatitis B:* Transmission occurs during contact with infected body fluids, such as blood, semen, saliva, and vaginal secretions. Infection causes increased risk of fulminant hepatitis, chronic infection, and subsequent cirrhosis and hepatocellular carcinoma. Adults between 20 and 39 years of age are most affected, especially injection drug users and sex workers. Provide behavioral counseling and serologic screening for patients at risk. Hepatitis B vaccine is recommended for all young adults not previously immunized, injection drug users and their sexual partners, people at risk for sexually transmitted diseases, travelers to endemic areas, recipients of blood products as in hemodialysis, and health care workers with frequent exposure to blood products. Many of these groups also should be screened for HIV infection.

■ *Hepatitis C:* Hepatitis C, now the most common form, is spread by blood exposure and is associated with injection drug use. No vaccine is available.

*U.S. Preventive Services Task Force: Guide to Clinical Preventive Services (2nd ed.). Baltimore, Williams & Wilkins, p. 572, 1996.

For colorectal cancer, screen for risk factors, namely family history of colonic polyps, history of colorectal cancer or adenoma in a first-degree relative, and personal history of ulcerative colitis, adenomatous polyps, or prior diagnosis of endometrial, ovarian, or breast cancer. Consider annual testing with the fecal occult blood test (FOBT), colonoscopy, or both for all people older than 50 years.*
Detection rates for colorectal cancer and insertion depths of endoscopy are roughly as follows: 25% to 30% at 20 cm; 50% to 55% at 35 cm; 40% to 65% at 40 cm to 50 cm. Full colonoscopy or air contrast barium enema detects 80% to 95% of colorectal cancers, but is uncomfortable and expensive.

TECHNIQUES   **POSSIBLE FINDINGS**

TECHNIQUES OF EXAMINATION

THE ABDOMEN

○— **Inspect** the abdomen, including

■ Skin	Scars, striae, veins
■ Umbilicus	Hernia, inflammation
■ Contours for shape, symmetry, enlarged organs or masses	Bulging flanks, suprapubic bulge, large liver or spleen, tumors
■ Any peristaltic waves	GI obstruction
■ Any pulsations	Increased in aortic aneurysm

Auscultate the abdomen for

■ Bowel sounds	Increased or decreased motility
■ Bruits	Bruit of renal artery stenosis

---

*U.S. Preventive Services Task Force: Guide to Clinical Preventive Services (2nd ed.). Baltimore, Williams & Wilkins, p. 572, 1996.

TECHNIQUES	POSSIBLE FINDINGS

Bowel Sounds and Bruits

Change	Seen With
Increased bowel sounds	Diarrhea Early intestinal obstruction
Decreased, then absent bowel sounds	Adynamic ileus Peritonitis
High-pitched, tinkling bowel sounds	Intestinal fluid Air under tension in a dilated bowel
High-pitched, rushing bowel sounds	Intestinal obstruction
Hepatic bruit	Carcinoma of the liver Alcoholic hepatitis
Arterial bruit	Partial obstruction of the aorta or renal arteries

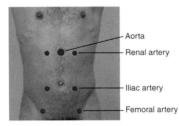

- Aorta
- Renal artery
- Iliac artery
- Femoral artery

■ Friction rubs	Liver tumor, splenic infarct
Percuss the abdomen for patterns of tympany and dullness.	Ascites, GI obstruction, pregnant uterus, ovarian tumor
Palpate all quadrants of the abdomen	

TECHNIQUES	POSSIBLE FINDINGS

■ Lightly for guarding, rebound, and tenderness

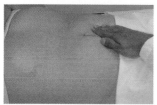

Peritoneal inflammation

■ Deeply for masses or tenderness

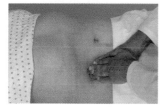

Tumors, a distended viscus

THE LIVER

Percuss span of liver dullness in the midclavicular line (MCL).

Hepatomegaly

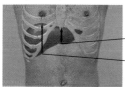

4 – 8 cm in midsternal line

6 – 12 cm in right midclavicular line

NORMAL LIVER SPANS

Feel the liver edge, if possible, as patient breathes in.

Firm edge of cirrhosis

TECHNIQUES	POSSIBLE FINDINGS

Measure its distance from the costal margin in the MCL.

Increased in hepatomegaly

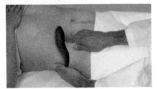 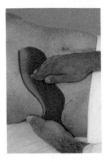

Note any tenderness or masses.

Tender liver of hepatitis or congestive heart failure; tumor mass

THE SPLEEN

Percuss across left lower anterior chest, noting change from tympany to dullness.

Check for a splenic percussion sign.

Try to **feel** spleen with the patient

Splenomegaly

■ Supine

■ ⌒⊦ Lying on the right side with legs flexed at hips and knees

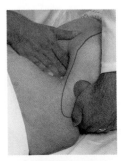

| **TECHNIQUES** | **POSSIBLE FINDINGS** |

THE KIDNEYS

Try to **palpate** each kidney.

Enlargement from cysts, cancer, hydronephrosis

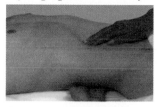

Check for costovertebral angle (CVA) tenderness.

Tender in kidney infection

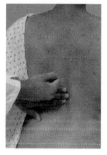

THE AORTA

Palpate the aorta's pulsations. In older people, also **estimate** its width.

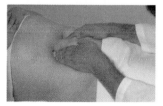

TECHNIQUES	POSSIBLE FINDINGS

SPECIAL TECHNIQUES

ASSESSING THE ACUTE ABDOMEN

Apply **light** and **deep palpation.**

Firm boardlike abdominal wall suggests peritoneal inflammation. *Guarding* occurs when the patient flinches, grimaces, or reports pain during palpation.

Check for *rebound tenderness,* pain that is greater when you withdraw your hand than when you press down. Press slowly on a tender area, then quickly "let go."

Rebound tenderness suggests peritoneal inflammation.

ASSESSING POSSIBLE APPENDICITIS

Follow the basic approach:

In classic appendicitis:

"Where did the pain begin?"

Near the umbilicus

"Where is it now?"

Right lower quadrant (RLQ)

Ask patient to cough: "Where does it hurt?"

RLQ

Search for local tenderness.

RLQ tenderness

Feel for muscular rigidity.

RLQ rigidity

Perform a rectal examination and, in women, a pelvic examination (see Chaps. 11 and 13).

Local tenderness, especially if appendix is retrocecal

■ *Rovsing's sign:* Press deeply and evenly in the *left* lower quadrant. Then quickly withdraw your fingers.

Pain in the *right* lower quadrant during *left*-sided pressure suggests appendicitis (a *positive* Rovsing's sign).

TECHNIQUES	POSSIBLE FINDINGS
■ *Psoas sign:* Place your hand just above the patient's right knee. Ask the patient to raise that thigh against your hand and to turn onto the left side. Then extend the patient's right leg at the hip to stretch the psoas muscle.	Pain from irritation of the psoas muscle suggests an inflamed appendix (a *positive* psoas sign).
■ *Obturator sign:* Flex the patient's right thigh at the hip, with the knee bent, and rotate the leg internally at the hip, which stretches the internal obturator muscle.	Right hypogastric pain constitutes a *positive* obturator sign, suggesting irritation of the obturator muscle by an inflamed appendix.

ASSESSING ACUTE CHOLECYSTITIS

Auscultate, percuss, and **palpate** the abdomen for tenderness.	Bowel sounds may be active or decreased; tympany may increase with an ileus; RUQ tenderness.
Assess for Murphy's sign. Hook your thumb under the right costal margin at edge of rectus muscle, and ask patient to take a deep breath.	Sharp tenderness and a sudden stop in inspiratory effort constitute a *positive* Murphy's sign.

ASSESSING PYELONEPHRITIS

Auscultate, percuss, and **palpate** the abdomen for tenderness.	Bowel sounds may be active or decreased. Tympany may be increased with an *ileus,* tenderness over the affected kidney.
Check for CVA tenderness on the posterior thorax.	Tenderness over inflamed kidney

TECHNIQUES	POSSIBLE FINDINGS

ASSESSING ASCITES

○—/○→ **Check** for shifting dullness. Map areas of tympany and dullness with patient supine and lying on side (see below).

Ascitic fluid usually shifts to dependent side, changing the margin of dullness (see below).

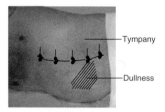

Tympany

Dullness

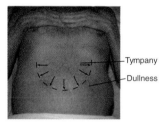

Tympany

Dullness

○— Check for a fluid wave. Ask patient or an assistant to press edges of both hands into midline of abdomen. Tap one side and feel for a wave transmitted to the other side.

A palpable wave suggests but does not prove ascites.

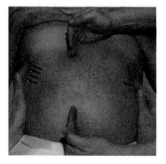

| TECHNIQUES | POSSIBLE FINDINGS |

○— **Ballotte** an organ or mass in an ascitic abdomen. Place your stiffened and straightened fingers on the abdomen, briefly jab them toward the structure, and try to touch its surface.

Your hand, quickly displacing the fluid, stops abruptly as it touches the solid surface.

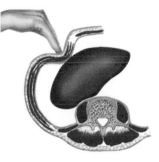

Recording the Physical Examination—The Abdomen

"Abdomen is protuberant with active bowel sounds. It is soft and nontender; no masses or hepatosplenomegaly. Liver span is 7 cm and in the right MCL; edge is smooth and palpable 1 cm below the right costal margin. Spleen and kidneys not felt. No CVA tenderness."

OR

"Abdomen is flat. No bowel sounds heard. It is firm and boardlike, with increased tenderness, guarding, and rebound in the right midquadrant. Liver percusses to 7 cm in the MCL; edge not felt. Spleen and kidneys not felt. No CVA tenderness."

Suggests peritonitis from possible appendicitis (see pp. 160–161)

AIDS TO INTERPRETATION

TABLE 9-1 ■ Diarrhea

Problem	Process	Characteristics of Stool
Acute Diarrhea		
Secretory Infections	Infection by viruses, preformed bacterial toxins (such as *Staphylococcus aureus, Clostridium perfringens,* toxigenic *Escherichia coli, Vibrio cholerae*), cryptosporidium, *Giardia lamblia*	Watery, without blood, pus, or mucus
Inflammatory Infections	Colonization or invasion of intestinal mucosa (nontyphoid *Salmonella, Shigella, Yersinia, Campylobacter,* enteropathic *E. coli, Entamoeba histolytica*)	Loose to watery, often with blood, pus, or mucus
Drug-Induced Diarrhea	Action of many drugs, such as magnesium-containing antacids, antibiotics, antineoplastic agents, and laxatives	Loose to watery

(table continues next page)

TABLE 9-1 ■ Diarrhea *(Continued)*

Problem	Process	Characteristics of Stool
Chronic Diarrhea		
Diarrheal Syndromes		
■ Irritable bowel syndrome	A disorder of bowel motility with alternating diarrhea and constipation	Loose; may show mucus but no blood. Small, hard stools with constipation
■ Cancer of the sigmoid colon	Partial obstruction by a malignant neoplasm	May be blood-streaked
Inflammatory Bowel Disease		
■ Ulcerative colitis	Inflammation of the mucosa and submucosa of the rectum and colon with ulceration; cause unknown	From soft to watery, often containing blood
■ Crohn's disease of the small bowel (regional enteritis) or colon (granulomatous colitis)	Chronic inflammation of the bowel wall, typically involving the terminal ileum, proximal colon, or both	Small, soft to loose or watery, usually free of gross blood (enteritis) or with less bleeding than ulcerative colitis (colitis)
Voluminous Diarrheas		
■ Malabsorption syndromes	Defective absorption of fat, including fat-soluble vitamins, with steatorrhea (excessive	Typically bulky, soft, light yellow to gray, mushy, greasy or oily, and sometimes frothy; particularly foul-

(table continues next page)

TABLE 9-1 ■ Diarrhea *(Continued)*		
Problem	**Process**	**Characteristics of Stool**
	excretion of fat) as in pancreatic insufficiency, bile salt deficiency, bacterial overgrowth	smelling; usually floats in the toilet
■ Osmotic diarrheas Lactose intolerance	Deficiency in intestinal lactase	Watery diarrhea of large volume
Abuse of osmotic purgatives	Laxative habit, often surreptitious	Watery diarrhea of large volume
■ Secretory diarrheas from bacterial infection, secreting villous adenoma, fat or bile salt malabsorption, hormone-mediated conditions (gastrin in Zollinger–Ellison syndrome, vasoactive intestinal peptide [VIP])	Variable	Watery diarrhea of large volume

TABLE 9-2 ■ Urinary Incontinence*

Problem	Mechanisms
Stress Incontinence	
The urethral sphincter is weakened so that transient increases in intra-abdominal pressure raise the bladder pressure to levels exceeding urethral resistance. This leads to voiding *small amounts* during laughing, coughing, and sneezing.	In women, weakness of the pelvic floor with inadequate muscular support of the bladder and proximal urethra and a change in the angle between the bladder and the urethra from childbirth, surgery, and local conditions affecting the internal urethral sphincter, such as postmenopausal atrophy of the mucosa and urethral infection In men, prostatic surgery
Urge Incontinence	
Detrusor contractions are stronger than normal and overcome the normal urethral resistance. The bladder is typically small. Results are voiding *moderate amounts,* urgency, frequency, and nocturia.	■ Decreased cortical inhibition of detrusor contractions, as from stroke, brain tumor, dementia, and lesions of the spinal cord above the sacral level ■ Hyperexcitability of sensory pathways, as from bladder infection, tumor, and fecal impaction ■ Deconditioning of voiding reflexes, caused by frequent voluntary voiding at low bladder volumes
Overflow Incontinence	
Detrusor contractions are insufficient to overcome urethral resistance. The bladder is typically large, even after an effort to void, leading to *continuous dribbling*.	■ Obstruction of the bladder outlet, as by benign prostatic hyperplasia or tumor

(table continues next page)

TABLE 9-2 ■ Urinary Incontinence* (Continued)

Problem	Mechanisms
	■ Weakness of the detrusor muscle associated with peripheral nerve disease at the sacral level ■ Impaired bladder sensation that interrupts the reflex arc, as from diabetic neuropathy
Functional Incontinence This is a functional inability to get to the toilet in time because of impaired health or environmental conditions.	Problems in mobility from weakness, arthritis, poor vision, other conditions; environmental factors such as an unfamiliar setting, distant bathroom facilities, bedrails, physical restraints
Incontinence Secondary to Medications Drugs may contribute to any type of incontinence listed.	Sedatives, tranquilizers, anticholinergics, sympathetic blockers, potent diuretics

*Patients may have more than one kind of incontinence.

TABLE 9-3 ■ Tender Abdomens

Visceral Tenderness	Peritoneal Tenderness

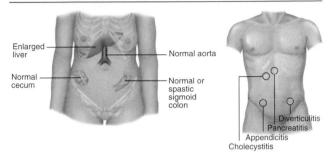

Enlarged liver

Normal cecum

Normal aorta

Normal or spastic sigmoid colon

Diverticulitis
Pancreatitis
Appendicitis
Cholecystitis

Tenderness From Disease in the Chest and Pelvis

Acute Pleurisy	*Acute Salpingitis*

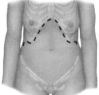

Unilateral or bilateral, upper or lower abdom

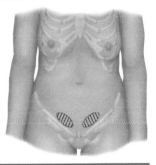

The Male Genitalia

THE HEALTH HISTORY

Common or Concerning Symptoms

- Sexual function, sexual preference
- Penile discharge or lesions
- Scrotal pain, swelling, or lesions

Pose general questions such as "How is sexual function for you?" "Are you satisfied with your sexual life?" "What about your ability to perform sexually?" Ask if desire for or level of sexual activity has changed any in recent years.

To assess *libido*, or desire, ask, "Have you maintained an interest in sex?"

Decreased interest from psychogenic causes such as depression, endocrine dysfunction, or side effects of medications

For the *arousal* phase, ask "Can you achieve and maintain an erection?"

Erectile dysfunction from psychogenic causes, especially if early morning erection is preserved; also from decreased testosterone, decreased blood flow in hypogastric arterial system, impaired neural innervation

If *ejaculation* is premature, or early and out of control, ask "About how long does intercourse last?" "Do you climax too soon?" For reduced or absent ejaculation, "Do you find that you cannot have orgasm even though you can have an erection?" Try to determine if the problem involves the pleasurable sensation of *orgasm,* the ejaculation of seminal fluid, or both.

Premature ejaculation is common, especially in young men. Less common is reduced or absent ejaculation affecting middle-aged or older men. Possible causes are medications, surgery, neurologic deficits, or lack of androgen. Lack of orgasm with ejaculation is usually psychogenic.

To assess the possibility of genital infection from sexually transmitted diseases (STDs), ask about any *discharge from the penis.*

Penile discharge in gonococcal (usually yellow) and nongonococcal (clear or white) urethritis

Inquire about *sores or growths on the penis* and any *pain or swelling in the scrotum.*

See Table 10-1, Abnormalities of the Penis (pp. 177–178) and Table 10-2, Abnormalities of the Male Genitalia (pp. 178–180).

Because STDs may involve other parts of the body, additional questions about oral and anal sex are often indicated. If the patient engages in these practices, ask also about sore throat, diarrhea, rectal bleeding, and oral itching or pain.

HEALTH PROMOTION AND COUNSELING

Important Topics for Health Promotion and Counseling

- Prevention of STDs and HIV
- Testicular self-examination

Focus on patient education about STDs and HIV, early detection of infection during history taking and physical examination, and identification and treatment of infected partners. Identify the patient's sexual orientation, the number of sexual partners in the past month, and any history of STDs. Also query use of alcohol and drugs, particularly injection drugs. Counsel patients at risk about limiting the number of partners, using condoms, and establishing regular medical care for treatment of STDs and HIV.

Counseling and testing for HIV is recommended for all people at increased risk for infection with HIV, STDs, or both; men with male partners; past or present injection drug users; any past or present partners of people with HIV infection, bisexual practices, or injection drug use; and patients with a history of transfusion between 1978 and 1985.

Encourage men, especially those between 15 and 35 years of age, to perform monthly testicular self-examinations.

PATIENT INSTRUCTIONS FOR THE
TESTICULAR SELF-EXAMINATION

This examination is best performed after a warm bath or shower. The heat relaxes the scrotum and makes it easier to find anything unusual.

- Standing in front of a mirror, check for any swelling on the skin of the scrotum.
- Examine each testicle with both hands. Cup the index and middle fingers under the testicle and place the thumbs on top.
- Roll the testicle gently between the thumbs and fingers. One testicle may be larger than the other . . . that's normal, but be concerned about any lump or area of pain.
- Find the epididymis. This is a soft, tubelike structure at the back of the testicle that collects and carries sperm, not an abnormal lump.

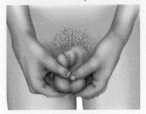

- If you find any lump, don't wait. See your doctor. The lump may just be an infection, but if it is cancer, it will spread unless stopped by treatment.

(*Adapted from the National Cancer Institute. Rex.nih.gov/WINK PUBS/testicular/testexam.htm. Accessed 9/27/01.)

TECHNIQUES	POSSIBLE FINDINGS

TECHNIQUES OF EXAMINATION

■ Male Genitalia

This examination usually is deferred until the patient is standing.

Wear gloves.

∘— THE PENIS

Inspect the

■ Development of the penis and the skin and hair at its base	Sexual maturation, lice
■ Prepuce	Phimosis
■ Glans	Balanitis, chancre, herpes, warts, cancer
■ Urethral meatus	Hypospadias, discharge of urethritis

Palpate

■ Any visible lesions	Chancre, cancer
■ The shaft	Urethral stricture or cancer

THE SCROTUM AND ITS CONTENTS

Inspect

■ Contours of scrotum	Hernia, hydrocele, cryptorchidism

TECHNIQUES	POSSIBLE FINDINGS
■ Skin of scrotum	Rashes
Palpate each	
■ Testis, noting any	
■ Lumps	Cancer
■ Tenderness	Orchitis, torsion
■ Epididymis	Epididymitis, cyst
■ Spermatic cord and adjacent areas	Varicocele

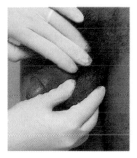 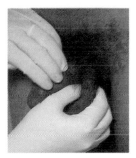

■ Hernias

Inspect inguinal and femoral areas as patient strains down.	Inguinal and femoral hernias

TECHNIQUES	**POSSIBLE FINDINGS**
Palpate external inguinal ring through scrotal skin and ask patient to strain down.	Indirect and direct inguinal hernias

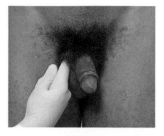

Recording the Physical Examination—Male Genitalia and Hernias

"Circumcised male. No penile discharge or lesions. No scrotal swelling or discoloration. Testes descended bilaterally, smooth, without masses. Epididymis nontender. No inguinal or femoral hernias."

OR

"Uncircumcised male; prepuce easily retractible. No penile discharge or lesions. No scrotal swelling or discoloration. Testes descended bilaterally; right testicle smooth; 1 × 1 cm firm nodule on left lateral testicle. It is fixed and nontender. Epididymis nontender. No inguinal or femoral hernias."

Suspicious for testicular carcinoma, the most common form of cancer in men between 15 and 35 years of age

AIDS TO INTERPRETATION

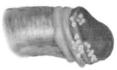

TABLE 10-1 ■ Abnormalities of the Penis

Venereal Wart

Warty growths on the glans, shaft, or base of penis; caused by human papillomavirus

Genital Herpes

A cluster of small vesicles, typically on the glans, that evolves into painful, small ulcers on red bases

Syphilitic Chancre

A usually nontender, firm erosion or ulcer, typically on the glans; caused by primary syphilis

Hypospadias

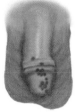

Congenital displacement of the urethral meatus to the inferior surface of the penis

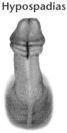

(table continues next page)

TABLE 10-1 ■ Abnormalities of the Penis *(Continued)*

Peyronie's Disease

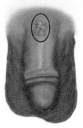

Palpable nontender hard plaques just beneath the skin, usually along the dorsum of the penis, leading to crooked, painful erections

Cancer of the Penis

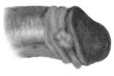

An indurated and usually nontender nodule or ulcer of the glans or inner surface of the prepuce; seen mainly in uncircumcised men

TABLE 10-2 ■ Abnormalities of the Male Genitalia

Hydrocele

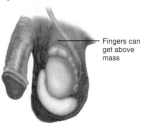

Fingers can get above mass

A fluid-filled sac in the tunica vaginalis. The clinician's fingers can get above the scrotal mass.

(table continues next page)

TABLE 10-2 ■ Abnormalities of the
Male Genitalia *(Continued)*

Scrotal Hernia

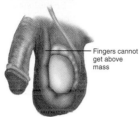

Fingers cannot get above mass

Protrusion of abdominal contents through the external inguinal ring into the scrotum. The clinician's fingers cannot get above the mass.

Acute Orchitis

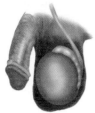

An acutely tender, swollen testis from infection

Acute Epididymitis

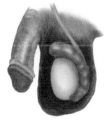

A tender, swollen epididymis, usually associated with infection of the urinary tract or prostate

Varicocele

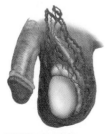

Varicose veins of the spermatic cord, traditionally described as feeling like a "bag of worms"

(table continues next page)

TABLE 10-2 ■ Abnormalities of the
Male Genitalia (Continued)

Small Testis

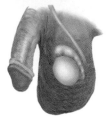

Small, firm testes suggest Klinefelter's syndrome; small, soft testis(es) suggest atrophy.

Cryptorchidism

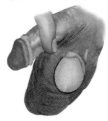

An undescended testicle, not palpable in the scrotum. The scrotal sac is poorly developed on the involved side(s). Associated with increased risk of testicular carcinoma.

Testicular Carcinoma

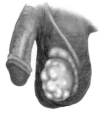

A usually painless, solid nodule or mass in the testis

Torsion of the Spermatic Cord

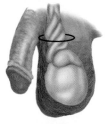

An acutely tender, swollen testis due to twisting of the organ on the spermatic cord, with resulting circulatory impairment

TABLE 10-3 ■ Hernias in the Groin

Indirect Inguinal

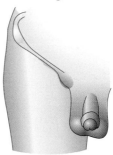

Most common hernia at all ages, both sexes. Originates above inguinal ligament and often passes into scrotum. *May touch examiner's fingertip in inguinal canal.*

Direct Inguinal

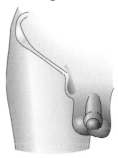

Less common than indirect hernia, usually occurs in men older than 40 years. Originates above inguinal ligament near external inguinal ring and *rarely enters scrotum. May bulge anteriorly, touching side of examiner's finger.*

Femoral

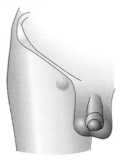

Least common hernia, more common in women than in men. Originates below inguinal ligament, more lateral than inguinal hernia. *Never enters scrotum.*

The Female Genitalia

THE HEALTH HISTORY

Common or Concerning Symptoms

- Menstrual history, menopause
- Pregnancy
- Vulvovaginal symptoms
- Sexual activity

For the *menstrual history,* ask the patient how old she was when her monthly, or menstrual, periods began (age at menarche). When did her last period start, and, if possible, the one before that? How often do the periods come (as measured by the intervals between the first days of successive periods)? How regular or irregular are they? How long do they last? How heavy is the flow?

The dates of previous periods may alert you to possible pregnancy or menstrual irregularities.

Menopause, the absence of menses for 12 consecutive months, usually occurs between 45 and 52 years of age. Associated symptoms

Postmenopausal bleeding raises the question of endometrial cancer.

include hot flashes, flushing, sweating, and sleep disturbances. *Postmenopausal bleeding* is defined as bleeding that occurs after 6 months without periods and warrants further investigation.

Amenorrhea refers to the absence of periods. Failure to begin periods is called *primary amenorrhea,* while cessation of periods after their establishment is termed *secondary amenorrhea.*

Secondary amenorrhea from low body weight related to any cause, including malnutrition, anorexia nervosa, stress, chronic illness, and hypothalamic–pituitary–ovarian dysfunction

If amenorrhea suggests a *current pregnancy,* inquire about history of intercourse and *common early symptoms:* tenderness, tingling, or increased size of breasts; urinary frequency; nausea and vomiting; easy fatigability; and feelings that the baby is moving (usually noted at about 20 weeks).

Amenorrhea followed by heavy bleeding suggests a threatened abortion or dysfunctional uterine bleeding.

For *vaginal discharge* and local *itching,* inquire about amount, color, consistency, and odor of discharge.

See Table 11-1, Lesions of the Vulva, pp. 191–192; also Table 11-4, Vaginitis, p. 195.

To assess sexual function, start with general questions such as "How is sex for you?" Or "Are you having any problems with sex?"

Direct questions help you assess each phase of the sexual response: desire, arousal, and orgasm.

Ask also about *dyspareunia,* or discomfort or pain during intercourse.

Superficial pain suggests local inflammation, atrophic vaginitis, or inadequate lubrication; deeper pain may result from pelvic disorders or pressure on a normal ovary.

For *sexually transmitted diseases* (STDs), identify the preference as to sexual partners (male, female, or both) and the number of sexual partners in the previous month. Ask if the patient has concerns about HIV infection, desires HIV testing, or has current or past partners at risk.

HEALTH PROMOTION AND COUNSELING

Important Topics for Health Promotion and Counseling

- Pap smear screening
- Options for family planning
- STDs and HIV
- Changes in menopause

Pap smear screening should begin at 18 years of age or with onset of sexual activity. Annual testing until 65 years of age has been common but does not appear to improve detection compared to longer intervals. Several professional organizations recommend annual Pap smears for 3 years and then, if results are normal, less frequently based on clinician discretion. Perform Pap smears more frequently for women at increased risk—those with early onset of sexual activity, multiple partners, infection with human papillomavirus or HIV, or limited access to regular medical care.

Counsel women, particularly adolescents, about the *timing of ovulation* in the menstrual cycle and how to plan or prevent pregnancy. Discuss methods for family planning and their effectiveness: natural (periodic abstinence, withdrawal, lactation); barrier (condom, diaphragm, cervical cap); implantable (intrauterine device, subdermal implant); pharmacologic (spermicide, oral contraceptives, subdermal implant of levonorgesterel, estrogen/progesterone injectables); and surgical (tubal ligation).

For STDs and HIV, assess risk factors for infection by taking a careful sexual history and counseling patients about spread of disease and ways to reduce high-risk practices.

Be familiar with the psychological and physiologic changes of *menopause.* Help the patient to weigh the benefits and risks of treatment, taking into account the personal and family history of cardiovascular disease and osteoporosis.

TECHNIQUES OF EXAMINATION

TIPS FOR THE SUCCESSFUL PELVIC EXAMINATION

The Patient	The Examiner
■ Avoids intercourse, douching, or use of vaginal suppositories for 24 to 48 hours before examination ■ Empties bladder before examination ■ Lies supine, with head and shoulders slightly elevated, arms at sides or folded across chest to reduce tightening of abdominal muscles	■ Explains each step of the examination in advance ■ Drapes patient from mid-abdomen to knees; depresses drape between knees to provide eye contact with patient ■ Avoids unexpected or sudden movements ■ Warms speculum with tap water ■ Monitors comfort of the examination by watching the patient's face ■ Uses excellent but gentle technique, especially when inserting the speculum

TECHNIQUES	POSSIBLE FINDINGS

Wear gloves.

EXTERNAL GENITALIA

○— **Observe** pubic hair to assess sexual maturity.

Normal or delayed puberty

∿ **Inspect** the external genitalia.

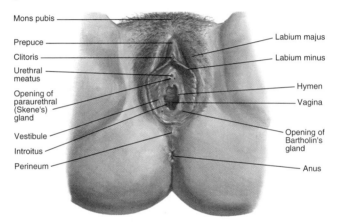

Mons pubis
Prepuce
Clitoris
Urethral meatus
Opening of paraurethral (Skene's) gland
Vestibule
Introitus
Perineum

Labium majus
Labium minus
Hymen
Vagina
Opening of Bartholin's gland
Anus

- Labia

Inflammation

- Clitoris

Enlarged in masculinization

- Urethral orifice

Urethral caruncle

- Introitus

Imperforate hymen

Palpate for enlargement or tenderness of Bartholin's glands.

Bartholin's gland infection

Milk the urethra for discharge, if indicated.

Discharge of urethritis

TECHNIQUES	POSSIBLE FINDINGS

INTERNAL GENITALIA AND PAP SMEAR

Locate the cervix with a gloved and water-lubricated index finger.

Assess support of vaginal outlet by asking patient to strain down.

Cystocele, cystourethrocele, rectocele

Enlarge the introitus by pressing its posterior margin downward.

Insert a water-lubricated speculum of suitable size, starting with speculum held obliquely.

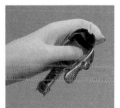

ENTRY ANGLE

Rotate speculum, open it and inspect cervix.

Observe

■ Position

Cervix faces forward if uterus is retroverted.

■ Color

Purplish in pregnancy

TECHNIQUES	POSSIBLE FINDINGS
■ Epithelial surface	Squamous and columnar epithelium

External os of the cervix
Columnar epithelium
Squamocolumnar junction
Transformation zone
Squamous epithelium

TECHNIQUES	POSSIBLE FINDINGS
■ Any discharge or bleeding	Discharge from os in mucopurulent cervicitis
■ Any ulcers, nodules, or masses	Herpes, polyp, cancer
Obtain specimens for cytology (Pap smears) with	Early cancer before it is clinically evident
■ An endocervical spatula or brush (except in pregnant women), to scrape the ectocervix	
■ Or, if the woman is not pregnant, a cervical broom for a combined specimen (also used for Thin Prep)	
Inspect the vaginal mucosa as you withdraw the speculum.	Bluish color and deep rugae in pregnancy; vaginal cancer
Palpate the cervix and fornices.	Pain on moving cervix in pelvic inflammatory disease

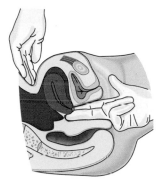

Palpate, by means of a bimanual examination,

■ The uterus

Pregnancy, myomas; soft isthmus in early pregnancy

■ Right and left adnexa

Ovarian masses, salpingitis, tubal pregnancy

Assess strength of pelvic muscles. With your vaginal fingers clear of the cervix, ask patient to tighten her muscles around your fingers as hard and long as she can.

A firm squeeze that compresses your fingers, moves them up and inward, and lasts more than 3 seconds is full strength.

♀ / ♂ **Perform** a rectovaginal examination (see Chap. 13).

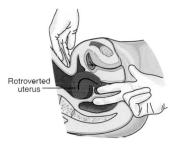

Rotroverted uterus

TECHNIQUES	POSSIBLE FINDINGS

SPECIAL TECHNIQUE

HERNIAS

Ask woman to strain down, as
you palpate for a bulge in

■ The femoral canal   Femoral hernia

■ The labia majora up to just   Indirect inguinal hernia
  lateral to the pubic tubercle

Recording the Physical Examination— Female Genitalia

"No inguinal adenopathy. External genitalia without
erythema or lesions; no lesions or masses. Vaginal mucosa
pink. Cervix parous, pink, and without discharge. Uterus
anterior, midline, smooth, and not enlarged. No adnexal
tenderness. Pap smear obtained. Rectovaginal wall intact."

AIDS TO INTERPRETATION

TABLE 11-1 ■ Lesions of the Vulva

Epidermoid Cyst

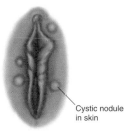

Cystic nodule
in skin

Small, firm, round cystic nodules in the labia suggest epidermoid cysts. They are sometimes yellowish in color. Look for the dark punctum marking the blocked opening of the gland.

Venereal Wart
(Condyloma Acuminatum)

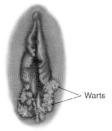

Warts

Warty lesions on the labia and within the vestibule suggest condylomata acuminata from infection with human papillomavirus.

Genital Herpes

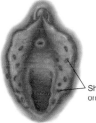

Shallow ulcers
on red bases

Shallow, small, painful ulcers on red bases suggest a herpes infection. Initial infection may be extensive, as illustrated here. Recurrent infections are usually confined to a small local patch.

(table continues next page)

TABLE 11-1 ■ Lesions of the Vulva *(Continued)*

Syphilitic Chancre

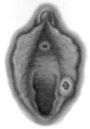

A firm, painless ulcer suggests the chancre of primary syphilis. Because most chancres in women develop internally, they often go undetected.

Secondary Syphilis
(Condyloma Latum)

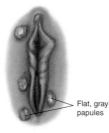

Flat, gray papules

Slightly raised, flat, round or oval papules covered by a gray exudate suggest condylomata lata. These constitute one manifestation of secondary syphilis and are contagious.

Carcinoma of the Vulva

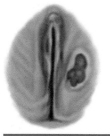

An ulcerated or raised red vulvar lesion in an elderly woman may indicate vulvar carcinoma.

TABLE 11-2 ■ Variations in the Cervix

Normal Variations

Oval

Slitlike

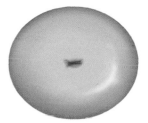

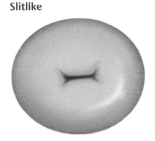

Lacerations

Unilateral Transverse

Bilateral Transverse

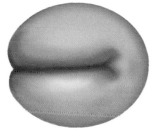

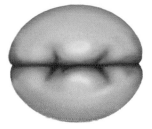

Stellate

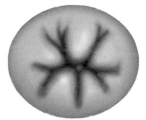

TABLE 11-3 ■ Abnormalities of the Cervix

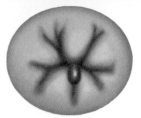

Endocervical polyp. A bright red, smooth mass that protrudes from the os suggests a polyp. It bleeds easily.

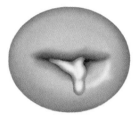

Mucopurulent cervicitis. A yellowish exudate emerging from the cervical os suggests this diagnosis. Causes include *Chlamydia* and gonococcal infections.

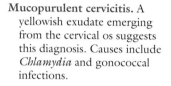

Carcinoma of the cervix. An irregular, hard mass suggests cancer. Early lesions cannot be detected by physical examination alone.

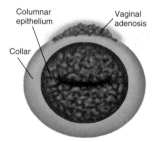

Columnar epithelium

Vaginal adenosis

Collar

Fetal exposure to diethylstilbestrol. Several changes may be seen: a color of tissue around the cervix, columnar epithelium that covers the cervix or extends to the vaginal wall (then termed *vaginal adenosis*), and, rarely, carcinoma of the vagina.

TABLE 11-4 ■ Vaginitis

	Discharge	Other Symptoms
Trichomonas vaginitis	Yellowish green, often profuse, may be malodorous	Itching, vaginal soreness, dyspareunia
Candida vaginitis	White, curdy, often thick, not malodorous	Itching, vaginal soreness, external dysuria, dyspareunia
Bacterial vaginosis	Gray or white, thin homogeneous, scant, malodorous	Fishy genital odor
Atrophic vaginitis	Variable in color, consistency, and amount; may be blood tinged; rarely profuse	Itching, dysuria, dyspareunia

Vulva	Vagina	Laboratory Assessment
May be red	May be normal or red, with red spots, petechiae	Saline wet mount for trichomonads
Often red and swollen	Often red with white patches of discharge	KOH preparation for branching hyphae
Usually normal	Usually normal	Saline wet mount for "clue cells," "whiff test" with KOH for fishy odor
Atrophic	Atrophic, dry, pale; may be red, petechial, ecchymotic; possible erosions or adhesions	

TABLE 11-5 ■ Relaxations of the Pelvic Floor

When the pelvic floor is weakened, various structures may become displaced. These displacements are seen best when the patient strains down.

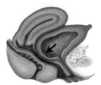

A **cystocele** is a bulge of the anterior wall of the upper part of the vagina, together with the urinary bladder above it.

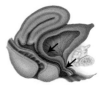

A **cystourethrocele** involves both the bladder and the urethra as they bulge into the anterior vaginal wall throughout most of its extent.

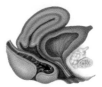

A **rectocele** is a bulge of the posterior vaginal wall, together with a portion of the rectum.

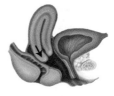

A **prolapsed uterus** has descended down the vaginal canal. There are three degrees of severity: first, still within the vagina (as illustrated); second, with the cervix at the introitus; and third, with the cervix outside the introitus.

TABLE 11-6 ■ Positions of the Uterus and Uterine Myomas

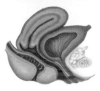

An anteverted uterus lies in a forward position at roughly a right angle to the vagina. This is the most common position. *Anteflexion*—a forward flexion of the uterine body in relation to the cervix—often coexists.

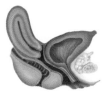

A retroverted uterus is tilted posteriorly with its cervix facing anteriorly.

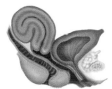

A retroflexed uterus has a posterior tilt that involves the uterine body but not the cervix. A uterus that is retroflexed or retroverted may be felt only through the rectal wall; some cannot be felt at all.

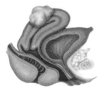

A myoma of the uterus is a very common, benign tumor that feels firm and often irregular. There may be more than one. A myoma on the posterior surface of the uterus may be mistaken for a retrodisplaced uterus; one on the anterior surface may be mistaken for an anteverted uterus.

The Pregnant Woman 12

THE HEALTH HISTORY

Common or Concerning Symptoms

- Symptoms of pregnancy
- Toxic exposures, use of illicit drugs, domestic violence
- Prior complications of pregnancy
- Chronic illnesses in patient or family members

During the initial visit, focus the history on the woman's *current state of health* and on risk factors for any conditions that could adversely affect her or the developing fetus. Ask about symptoms of pregnancy: breast tenderness, nausea or vomiting, urinary frequency, change in bowel habits, fatigue; her attitude toward the pregnancy, and if she plans to continue to term; eating patterns and quality of nutrition; tobacco, alcohol, and drug use; income and social support network; any exposure to teratogenic drugs or toxic substances; any history of domestic violence, which may escalate during pregnancy; *prior pregnancies,* because past obstetric problems tend to recur; major complications; *past medical history,* especially any chronic diseases such as hypertension, diabetes, or cardiac conditions; and *family history* for these conditions.

Calculate the *expected weeks of gestation by dates:* counted in weeks from either (1) the first day of the last menstrual period (*LMP*), known as *menstrual age,* or (2) the date of conception, if this is known (*conception age*).

Calculate the *expected date of confinement (EDC)* by adding 7 days to the first day of the LMP, subtracting 3 months, and adding 1 year (*Nägele's rule*). For example, the first day of a patient's LMP was October 7, 2002. Her EDC would be July 14, 2003.

Estimate the expected size of the uterus before examining the woman. Compare the expected size by dates with what you actually palpate during bimanual examination (or abdominally if pregnancy is beyond 14 weeks). If the woman does not remember her LMP or has irregular menstrual cycles, date the pregnancy by palpation and subsequent monitoring of the growth curve, along with the time of first fetal movements. In some cases, ultrasound is needed.

HEALTH PROMOTION AND COUNSELING

Important Topics for Health Promotion and Counseling

- Nutrition
- Weight gain
- Exercise
- Screening for domestic violence

Evaluate the woman's nutritional status, including a diet history, measurement of height and weight, and screening for anemia by checking the hematocrit. Develop a nutrition plan appropriate to the woman's cultural preferences. Advocate a balanced increase in calories and protein, because protein will be used for energy rather than growth unless the woman consumes sufficient calories. At each visit, monitor weight gain and review nutritional goals for women at risk.

According to the American College of Obstetrics and Gynecology, in the absence of obstetric or medical complications, most women can perform moderate exercise to maintain cardiorespiratory and muscular fitness throughout pregnancy and the postpartum period. Women who have exercised regularly before pregnancy can continue mild to moderate exercise, preferably for short periods three times a week. Women starting exercise during pregnancy should be more cautious. After the first trimester, women should avoid exercise in the supine position, which can compress the inferior vena cava and decrease blood flow to the placenta.

Abuse in pregnancy, which may result in feticide, ranges from 8% to 22%. Prior patterns of abuse may intensify, increasing risks for miscarriage, low birth-weight baby, and late prenatal care. Direct nonjudgmental questioning in a private setting is recommended at each prenatal visit. Validate positive responses, and mark the area of any injury on a body map. Above all, ask the woman how you might help her. Offer information on safe shelters, counseling centers, hotline telephone numbers, and other sources of help.*

PREPARING FOR THE EXAMINATION

Show respect for the woman's comfort and privacy, as well as for her individual needs and sensitivities. Ask her to gown with the opening in front to ease the examination of both breasts and the pregnant abdomen.

Positioning

- The semisitting position with the knees bent (see p. 203) affords the most comfort and protects abdominal organs and vessels from the weight of the gravid uterus.
- Prolonged periods of lying on the back should be avoided, so abdominal palpation should be efficient in time and results.
- The pelvic examination also should be relatively quick.

(continued)

---

*National Domestic Violence Hotline: 1-800-799-SAFE;
National Domestic Violence Resource Center: 1-800-537-2238

PREPARING FOR THE EXAMINATION (continued)

Equipment

- The examiner's hands should be warm and firm yet gentle in palpation. The fingers should be together and flat against the abdominal or pelvic tissue. Palpation should be smooth and continuous rather than kneading, using the more sensitive palmar surfaces of the ends of the fingers.
- You may need a speculum larger than the usual size. Because of the increased vascularity of the vaginal and cervical structures, insert and open the speculum gently to avoid tissue trauma and bleeding.
- Avoid the cervical brush for Pap smears, because it often causes bleeding. Use the Ayre wooden spatula, a cotton-tipped applicator, or both.

TECHNIQUES	POSSIBLE FINDINGS

TECHNIQUES OF EXAMINATION

GENERAL INSPECTION

Assess the woman's

- Overall health
- Nutritional status
- Neuromuscular coordination
- Emotional state

VITAL SIGNS AND WEIGHT

Take the blood pressure. In midpregnancy, it may be lower than in the nonpregnant state.	High blood pressure before 24 weeks indicates chronic hypertension. After 24 weeks, further evaluation is required to diagnose and to treat *pregnancy-induced hypertension (PIH).*

TECHNIQUES	POSSIBLE FINDINGS
Measure the weight. First-trimester weight loss should not exceed 5 pounds.	More than 5 pounds may be from excessive vomiting or *hyperemesis.*

HEAD AND NECK

Face. Check for the mask of pregnancy, *chloasma*, or irregular brownish patches around the eyes or across the bridge of the nose.	Facial edema after 24 weeks suggests PIH.
Hair	Localized patches of hair loss
Eyes. Note the conjunctival color.	Anemia of pregnancy may cause conjunctival pallor.
Nose, including nasal congestion	
Mouth	
Thyroid gland. Inspect and palpate. Symmetric enlargement is common.	Marked or asymmetric enlargement is not caused by pregnancy.

THORAX AND LUNGS

Inspect for the pattern of breathing.	Respiratory alkalosis in later trimesters

HEART

Palpate the apical impulse. It may be slightly higher than normal because of dextrorotation of the heart from the higher diaphragm.	
Auscultate the heart. Soft, blowing murmurs are common.	

BREASTS

Inspect the breasts and nipples for symmetry and color. The venous pattern may be marked, the nipples and areolae are dark, and Montgomery's glands are prominent.

Palpate for masses. During pregnancy, breasts are tender and nodular.

Compress each nipple between your index finger and thumb. This may express colostrums from the nipples.

ABDOMEN

Position the pregnant woman in a semi-sitting position with her knees flexed.

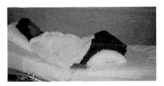

■ **Inspect** any scars or striae, the shape and contour of the abdomen, and the fundal height. Purplish striae and linea nigra are normal in pregnancy.

TECHNIQUES	POSSIBLE FINDINGS

■ **Assess** the shape and
contour to estimate
pregnancy size.

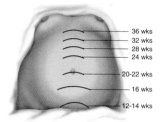

■ **Palpate** for:

Organs or masses

Fetal movements, usually
detected after 24 weeks

Uterine contractility

**EXPECTED HEIGHT OF THE
UTERINE FUNDUS BY MONTH
OF PREGNANCY**

Irregular contractions after
12 weeks or after palpation
during the third trimester
Before 37 weeks, regular
uterine contractions or
bleeding are abnormal,
suggesting preterm labor.

If the woman is more than
20 weeks pregnant, **measure
fundal height** with a tape
measure from the top of the
symphysis pubis to the top
of the uterine fundus. After
20 weeks, measurement in
centimeters should roughly
equal the weeks of gestation.

If fundal height is >2 cm
higher than expected,
consider multiple gestation,
a big baby, extra amniotic
fluid, or uterine myoma. If
it is more than 2 cm lower,
then consider missed
abortion, transverse lie,
growth retardation, or false
pregnancy.

Auscultate the fetal heart,
noting its rate (FHR),
location, and rhythm. Use
either:

■ A doptone—the FHR is
audible after 12 weeks.

■ A fetoscope—the FHR is
audible after 18 weeks.

Lack of an audible fetal
heart may indicate
pregnancy of fewer weeks
than expected, fetal demise,
or false pregnancy.

| TECHNIQUES | POSSIBLE FINDINGS |

RATE (FHR)

The *fetal heart rate* usually is in the 160s during early pregnancy, and then slows to the 120s to 140s near term. After 32 to 34 weeks, the FHR should increase with fetal movement.

An FHR that drops noticeably near term with fetal movement could indicate poor placental circulation.

■ From 12 to 18 weeks, listen in the midline of the lower abdomen.

■ After 28 weeks, listen over the fetal back or chest. Use modified *Leopold's maneuvers* to palpate the fetal head and back and identify where to listen.

LOCATION

Leopold's maneuvers are important adjuncts to palpation of the pregnant abdomen. They help determine:

Common deviations include *breech presentation* (fetal buttocks present at the outlet of the maternal pelvis) and absence of the presenting part well down into the maternal pelvis at term.

■ *Fetal lie,* or where the fetus lies in relation to the woman's back (longitudinal or transverse)

■ *Presentation,* or the end of the fetus that is presenting at the pelvic inlet (head or buttocks)

■ *Location of the fetal back*

TECHNIQUES	POSSIBLE FINDINGS

- *Engagement,* or how far the presenting part of the fetus has descended into the maternal pelvis

- *Estimated fetal weight*

First Maneuver (Upper Pole). Stand at the woman's side facing her head. Keep the fingers of both examining hands together. Palpate gently with the fingertips to determine what part of the fetus is in the upper pole of the uterine fundus.

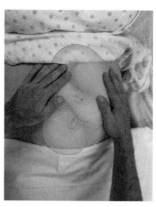

© B. Proud (photograph).

Second Maneuver (Sides of the Maternal Abdomen). Place one hand on each side of the woman's abdomen, aiming to capture the body of the fetus between them. Use one hand to steady the uterus and the other to palpate the fetus.

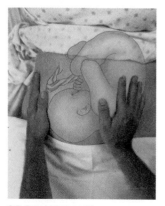

© B. Proud (photograph).

TECHNIQUES	**POSSIBLE FINDINGS**

Third Maneuver (Lower Pole). Face the woman's feet. Palpate the area just above the symphysis pubis. Note whether the hands diverge with downward pressure or stay together to learn if the presenting part of the fetus, head or buttocks, is descending into the pelvic inlet.

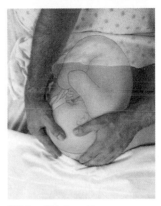

© B. Proud (photograph).

Fourth Maneuver (Confirmation of the Presenting Part). With your dominant hand grasp the part of the fetus in the lower pole, and with your nondominant hand, the part of the fetus in the upper pole. Try to distinguish between the head and the buttocks.

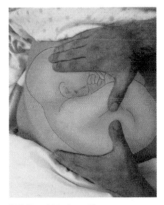

© B. Proud (photograph).

RHYTHM

In the third trimester, expect a variance of 10 to 15 beats per minute (BPM) over 1 to 2 minutes.

Lack of beat-to-beat variability late in pregnancy suggests fetal compromise.

TECHNIQUES	POSSIBLE FINDINGS

GENITALIA, ANUS, AND RECTUM

Inspect the *external genitalia*.

Parous relaxation of the introitus, enlargement of the labia and clitoris, scars from an *episiotomy* or perineal lacerations

Inspect the *anus*.

Hemorrhoids; may engorge later in pregnancy

Palpate *Bartholin's* and *Skene's glands*.

Check for a *cystocele* or *rectocele*.

Speculum Examination.
Inspect cervix for color, shape, and healed lacerations.

Purplish color of pregnancy; lacerations from prior deliveries

Take *Pap smears*, if indicated.

Vaginal infections (more common in pregnancy)

Inspect the *vaginal walls*.

Bluish or violet color, deep rugae, leukorrhea in normal pregnancy; vaginal irritation, itching, and discharge in infection

Bimanual Examination.
Insert two lubricated fingers into the introitus, palmar side down, with slight pressure downward on the perineum. Slide the fingers into the posterior vaginal vault. Maintaining downward pressure, gently turn the fingers palmar side up.

TECHNIQUES	POSSIBLE FINDINGS
■ **Assess** the cervical os and degree of effacement. Place your finger gently in the os, then sweep it around the *surface of the cervix.*	Closed os if nulliparous; os open to size of fingertip if multiparous
■ **Estimate** the *length of the cervix.* **Palpate** the lateral surface from the cervical tip to the lateral fornix.	Before 34 to 36 weeks, the cervix should retain its normal length of about 1.5 to 2 cm.
■ **Palpate** the *uterus* for size, shape, consistency, and position.	*Hegar's sign,* or early softening of the isthmus; pear-shaped uterus up to 8 weeks, then globular
■ **Estimate** *uterine size.* With your internal fingers placed at either side of the cervix, palmar surfaces upward, gently lift the uterus toward the abdominal hand. Capture the fundal portion of the uterus between your two hands and gently estimate size.	An irregularly shaped uterus suggests uterine myomata or a *bicornuate uterus,* two distinct uterine cavities separated by a septum.
■ **Palpate** the *left and right adnexa.*	Early in pregnancy, it is important to rule out tubal (*ectopic*) pregnancy.
■ **Perform** a *rectovaginal examination* to confirm uterine size or the integrity of the rectovaginal septum.	

TECHNIQUES	POSSIBLE FINDINGS

EXTREMITIES

Inspect the legs for *varicose veins.*

Inspect the hands and legs for *edema.*

Pathologic edema is often 3+ or more pretibially.

Obtain knee and ankle *reflexes.*

After 24 weeks, reflexes greater than 2+ may indicate PIH.

Recording the Physical Examination— The Pregnant Woman

"Abdomen: No surgical scars. Active bowel sounds. Soft, nontender; no palpable hepatosplenomegaly or masses. Fundus palpable 2 fingerbreadths below the umbilicus; shape is ovoid and smooth. Fetal heart rate 144. No inguinal adenopathy. External genitalia: midline episiotomy scar present. No lesions, discharge, or signs of infection. Bimanual examination: cervix midline, soft; external os admits fingertip, internal os closed. No pain elicited on movement of cervix; no adnexal masses. Fundus enlarged to 20 weeks' size, midline, smooth; vaginal tone reduced."

Describes examination of healthy pregnant woman at 20 weeks' gestation, third pregnancy

The Anus, Rectum, and Prostate

THE HEALTH HISTORY

Common or Concerning Symptoms

- Change in bowel habits
- Blood in the stool
- Pain with defecation, rectal bleeding, or tenderness
- Anal warts or fissures
- Weak stream of urine
- Burning with urination

In men, review the pattern of urination. Does the patient have any difficulty starting the urine stream or holding back urine? Is the flow weak? What about frequent urination, especially at night? Or pain or burning as he passes urine? Any blood in the urine or semen or pain with ejaculation? Is there frequent pain or stiffness in the lower back, hips, or upper thighs?

These symptoms suggest urethral obstruction as in benign prostatic hyperplasia or prostate cancer, especially in men older than 70 years.

HEALTH PROMOTION AND COUNSELING

Important Topics for Health Promotion and Counseling

- Screening for prostate cancer
- Screening for polyps and colorectal cancer

Prostate cancer is the leading cancer diagnosed in men in the United States and the second leading cause of death in North American men. Risk factors are age, family history of prostate cancer, and African American ethnicity. Screening methods such as the digital rectal examination (DRE) and the prostate-specific antigen (PSA) test are not highly accurate, which complicates decisions about screening of patients *without symptoms*. The DRE reaches only the posterior and lateral surfaces of the prostate, missing 25% to 35% of tumors in other areas. Sensitivity of the DRE for prostate cancer is low, ranging from 20% to 68%, and the rate of false positives is high. Recommendations about an annual DRE vary.

The benefits of PSA testing are also unclear. The PSA can be elevated in benign conditions like hyperplasia and prostatitis, and its detection rate for prostate cancer is low, about 28% to 35% in asymptomatic men. Several groups recommend annual combined screening with PSA and DRE for men older than 50 years and for African Americans and men older than 40 years with a positive family history.

For men *with symptoms* of prostate disorders, the clinician's role is more straightforward. Men with incomplete emptying of the bladder, urinary frequency or urgency, weak or intermittent stream or straining to initiate flow, hematuria, nocturia, or even bony pains in the pelvis should be encouraged to seek evaluation and treatment early.

To increase detection of colorectal cancer, both the DRE and the fecal occult blood test (FOBT) have significant limitations. The DRE permits the clinician to examine 7 to 8 cm of the rectum (usually about 11 cm long); only about 10% of colorectal cancers arise in this zone. The FOBT detects only 2% to 11% of colorectal cancers and 20% to 30% of adenomas in people older than 50 years. It results in a high rate of false positives. Among advocates, the DRE and FOBT usually are performed annually after 40 to 50 years of age. Recent recommendations favor a screening colonoscopy at 50 years of age, because flexible sigmoidoscopy permits good surveillance of only the distal third of the colon. Patients older than 40 years with familial polyposis, inflammatory bowel disease, or history of colon cancer in a first-degree relative should be advised to obtain a colonoscopy or air contrast barium enema every 3 to 5 years.

TECHNIQUES	POSSIBLE FINDINGS

TECHNIQUES OF EXAMINATION

Wear gloves.

MALE

Inspect the

■ Sacrococcygeal area	Pilonidal cyst or sinus
■ Perianal area	Hemorrhoids, warts, herpes, chancre, cancer

Palpate the anal canal and rectum with a lubricated and gloved finger. Feel the

TECHNIQUES	**POSSIBLE FINDINGS**

■ Walls of the rectum

Cancer of the rectum, polyps

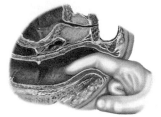

■ Prostate gland, as shown below

Benign hyperplasia, cancer, acute prostatitis

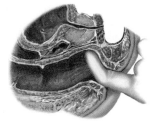

Try to **feel** above the prostate for irregularities or tenderness, if indicated.

Rectal shelf of peritoneal metastases; tenderness of inflammation

FEMALE

Inspect the anus.

Hemorrhoids

Palpate the anal canal and rectum.

Rectal cancer, normal uterine cervix or tampon (felt through the rectal wall)

Recording the Physical Examination—The Anus, Rectum, and Prostate

"No perirectal lesions or fissures. External sphincter tone intact. Rectal vault without masses. Prostate smooth and nontender with palpable median sulcus. (Or in a female, uterine cervix nontender.) Stool brown and hemoccult negative."

OR

"Perirectal area inflamed; no ulcerations, warts, or discharge. Cannot examine external sphincter, rectal vault, or prostate because of spasm of external sphincter and marked inflammation and tenderness of anal canal."

Raises concern of proctitis from infectious cause

OR

"No perirectal lesions or fissures. External sphincter tone intact. Rectal vault without masses. Left lateral prostate lobe with 1 × 1 cm firm hard nodule; right lateral lobe smooth; medial sulcus is obscured. Stool brown and hemoccult negative."

Raises concern of prostate cancer

AIDS TO INTERPRETATION

TABLE 13-1 ■ Abnormalities on Rectal Examination

External Hemorrhoids *(Thrombosed)*. Dilated hemorrhoidal veins that originate below the pectinate line, covered with skin; a tender, swollen, bluish ovoid mass is visible at the anal margin

Polyps of the Rectum. A soft mass that may or may not be on a stalk. May not be palpable.

Benign Prostatic Hyperplasia. An enlarged, nontender, smooth, firm but slightly elastic prostate gland; can cause symptoms without palpable enlargement

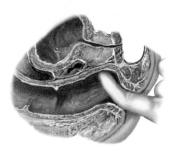

(table continues next page)

**TABLE 13-1 ■ Abnormalities on
Rectal Examination** *(Continued)*

Acute Prostatitis. A prostate
that is very tender, swollen
and firm because of acute
infection

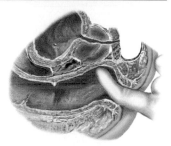

Cancer of the Prostate. A
hard area in the prostate
that may or may not feel
nodular

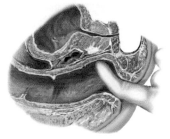

Cancer of the Rectum. Firm,
nodular, rolled edge of an
ulcerated cancer

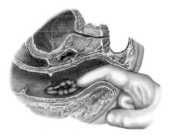

The Peripheral Vascular System

THE HEALTH HISTORY

Common or Concerning Symptoms

- Pain in the arms or legs
- Intermittent claudication
- Cold, numbness, pallor in the legs, hair loss
- Color change in fingertips or toes in cold weather
- Swelling in calves, legs, or feet
- Swelling with redness or tenderness

Begin by asking about any *pain in the arms and legs.*

To elicit symptoms of *arterial peripheral vascular disease* in the legs, inquire about *intermittent claudication,* exercise-induced pain that is absent at rest, makes the patient stop exertion, and abates within about 10 minutes. Ask, "Have you ever had any pain or cramping in your legs when you walk or exercise?" "How far can you walk without stopping to

Atherosclerosis can cause symptomatic limb ischemia with exertion; distinguish this from *spinal stenosis,* which produces leg pain with exertion that may be reduced by leaning forward (stretching the spinal cord in the narrowed vertebral canal) and less readily relieved by rest.

rest?" and "Does pain improve with rest?" Ask also about *coldness, numbness,* or *pallor* in legs or feet or *hair loss* over anterior tibial surfaces.

Hair loss over the anterior tibiae in decreased arterial perfusion. "Dry" or brown-black ulcers from gangrene may ensue.

Many patients have few symptoms, so identifying background risk factors (e.g., tobacco abuse, hypertension, diabetes, hyperlipidemia, and history of myocardial infarction or stroke) is important.

Only about 10% of affected patients have the classic symptoms of exertional calf pain relieved by rest.

To elicit symptoms of arterial spasm in the fingers or toes, ask "Do your fingertips ever change color in cold weather or when you handle cold objects?"

Digital ischemic changes of blanching, followed by cyanosis, then rubor with cold exposure and rewarming in Raynaud's phenomenon or disease.

Inquire about *venous peripheral vascular disease,* such as *swelling of feet and legs,* or any ulcers on lower legs, often the near ankles

Hyperpigmentation, edema, and possible cyanosis, especially when legs are dependent, in *venous stasis ulcers*

HEALTH PROMOTION AND COUNSELING

Important Topics for Health Promotion and Counseling

- Detection of peripheral arterial disease (PAD)
- Risk factors for PAD
- Screening for PAD: the ankle–brachial index (ABI)

Peripheral arterial disease (PAD) generally refers to atherosclerotic occlusion of arteries in the lower extremities. The femoral and popliteal arteries are involved most commonly, followed by the tibial and peroneal arteries. PAD affects from 12% to 25% of community populations; however, recent studies have shown that despite significant association with cardiovascular and cerebrovascular disease, PAD often is underdiagnosed in office practices. Most patients with PAD have either no symptoms or a range of *nonspecific leg symptoms,* such as *aching, cramping, numbness,* or *fatigue.*

Patients should be screened for subclinical PAD and targeted for aggressive risk factor intervention. Clinicians also should consider use of the ankle–brachial index (ABI), a highly accurate test for detecting stenoses of 50% or more in major vessels of the legs.

A wide range of interventions is available to reduce both onset and progression of subclinical PAD, including meticulous foot care and well-fitting shoes, tobacco cessation, treatment of hyperlipidemia, optimal control and treatment of diabetes and hypertension, use of antiplatelet agents, and, if needed, surgical revascularization.

TECHNIQUES OF EXAMINATION

Inspection of the limbs also may include findings relevant to the musculoskeletal and nervous systems.

TECHNIQUES	POSSIBLE FINDINGS

ARMS

Inspect for

■ Size and symmetry, any swelling

Lymphedema, venous obstruction

TECHNIQUES	POSSIBLE FINDINGS

- Venous pattern

  Venous obstruction

- Color and texture of skin and nails

  Raynaud's disease

Palpate and grade the pulses:

Grading Arterial Pulses	
4+	Bounding
3+	Increased
2+	Brisk, expected
1+	Diminished, weaker than expected
0	Absent, unable to palpate

- Radial

  Lost in thromboangiitis obliterans or acute arterial occlusion

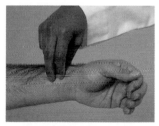

- Brachial

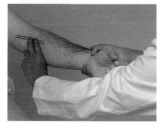

Feel for the epitrochlear nodes.

Lymphadenopathy from local cut, infection

| **TECHNIQUES** | **POSSIBLE FINDINGS** |

○— *LEGS*

Inspect for

- Size and symmetry, any swelling

  Venous insufficiency, lymphedema

- Venous pattern

  Varicose veins

- Color and texture of skin

  Pallor, rubor, cyanosis

- Hair distribution

  Loss in arterial insufficiency

Check for pitting edema.

Peripheral or systemic causes of edema

Palpate and grade the pulses:

Loss of pulses in acute arterial occlusion and arteriosclerosis obliterans

- Femoral

- Popliteal

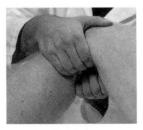

- Dorsalis pedis

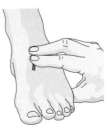

TECHNIQUES	**POSSIBLE FINDINGS**

■ Posterior tibial

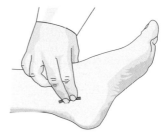

Lymphadenopathy

Palpate the inguinal lymph nodes:

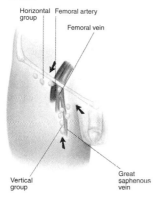

Horizontal group · Femoral artery · Femoral vein · Vertical group · Great saphenous vein

■ Horizontal group

■ Vertical group   Varicose veins

Ask patient to stand, and reinspect the venous pattern.

SPECIAL TECHNIQUE

Evaluating Arterial Supply to the Hand. Feel ulnar pulse, if possible. Perform an **Allen test**. Ask patient to

Persisting pallor of palm indicates occlusion of the released artery or its distal branches.

TECHNIQUES	POSSIBLE FINDINGS

SPECIAL TECHNIQUE

make a tight fist, palm up.
Occlude both radial and ulnar
arteries with your thumb. Ask
patient to open hand into a
relaxed, slightly flexed
position. Release your pressure
over one artery. Palm should
flush within about 3 to
5 seconds. Repeat, releasing
other artery.

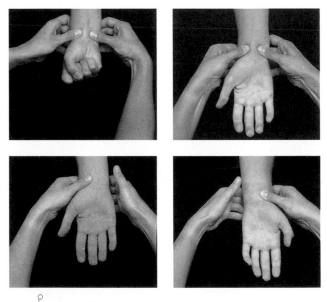

○— / ⌐**Postural Color
Changes of Chronic
Arterial Insufficiency.** Raise
both legs to approximately 60°
for about 1 minute. Then ask
patient to sit up with legs
dangling down. Note time

Marked pallor of feet on
elevation, delayed color return
and venous filling, and rubor
of dependent feet suggest
arterial insufficiency.

| TECHNIQUES | POSSIBLE FINDINGS |

SPECIAL TECHNIQUE

required for (1) return of pinkness, normally about 10 seconds or less, and (2) filling of veins on feet and ankles, normally about 15 seconds. Watch for development of any unusual rubor.

Recording the Physical Examination— The Peripheral Vascular System

"Extremities are warm and without edema. No varicosities or stasis changes. Calves are supple and nontender. No femoral or abdominal bruits. Brachial, radial, femoral, popliteal, dorsalis pedis (DP), and posterior tibial (PT) pulses are 2+ and symmetric."

OR

"Extremities are pale below the midcalf, with notable hair loss. Rubor noted when legs dependent but no edema or ulceration. Bilateral femoral bruits; no abdominal bruits heard. Brachial and radial pulses 2+; femoral, popliteal, DP, and PT pulses 1+." (Alternatively, pulses can be recorded as below.)

Suggests atherosclerotic PAD

	Radial	Brachial	Femoral	Popliteal	Dorsalis Pedis	Posterior Tibial
RT	2+	2+	1+	1+	1+	1+
LT	2+	2+	1+	1+	1+	1+

AIDS TO INTERPRETATION

TABLE 14-1 ■ Chronic Insufficiency of Arteries and Veins

Condition	Characteristics
Chronic Arterial Insufficiency 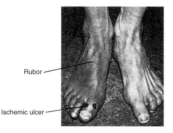 Rubor Ischemic ulcer	Intermittent claudication progressing to pain at rest. Decreased or absent pulses. Pale, especially on elevation; dusky red on dependency. Cool. No or mild edema, which may develop on lowering the leg to relieve pain. Thin, shiny, atrophic skin, with hair loss over foot and toes and thickened, ridged nails. Possible ulceration on toes or points of trauma on feet. Potential gangrene
Chronic Venous Insufficiency 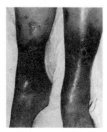	No to aching pain on dependency. Normal pulses, though may be hard to feel because of edema. Color normal or cyanotic on dependency; petechiae or brown pigment may develop. Often marked edema. Stasis dermatitis, possible thickening of skin, and narrowing of leg as scarring develops. Potential ulceration at sides of ankles. No gangrene.

TABLE 14-2 ■ Common Ulcers of the Feet and Ankles

Ulcer	Characteristics
Arterial Insufficiency 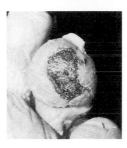	Located on toes, feet, or possible areas of trauma. No callus or excess pigment. May be atrophic. Pain often severe, unless masked by neuropathy. Possible gangrene. Decreased pulses, trophic changes, pallor of foot on elevation, dusky rubor on dependency.
Chronic Venous Insufficiency 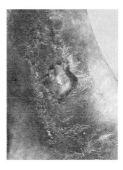	Located on inner or outer ankle. Pigmented, sometimes fibrotic. Pain not severe. No gangrene. Edema, pigmentation, stasis dermatitis, and possibly cyanosis of feet on dependency.
Neuropathic Ulcer 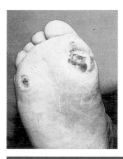	Located on pressure points in areas with diminished sensation, as in diabetic neuropathy. Skin calloused. No pain (which may cause ulcer to go unnoticed). Usually no gangrene. Decreased sensation, absent ankle jerks.

The Musculoskeletal System

FUNDAMENTALS FOR ASSESSING JOINTS

Assessing joints requires knowledge of their structure and function. Learn the surface landmarks and underlying anatomy of each major joint. Be familiar with the following terms:

- *Articular structures*—include the joint capsule and articular cartilage, synovium and synovial fluid, intra-articular ligaments, and juxta-articular bone

- *Nonarticular structures*—include periarticular ligaments, tendons, bursae, muscle, fascia, bone, nerve, and overlying skin

- *Ligaments*—the ropelike bundles of collagen fibrils that connect bone to bone

- *Tendons*—the collagen fibers that connect muscle to bone

- *Cartilage*—another type of collagen matrix

- *Bursae*—the pouches of synovial fluid that cushion the movement of tendons and muscles over bone or other joint structures

Review the three primary types of joint articulation—synovial, cartilaginous, and fibrous—and the varying degrees of movement each type allows.

Joints

Synovial Joints

- Freely movable
- Separated by **articular cartilage** and a **synovial cavity**
- Lubricated by synovial fluid
- Surrounded by a joint capsule

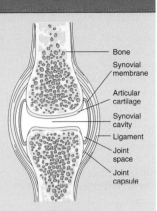

SYNOVIAL

Cartilaginous Joints

- Slightly movable
- Contain fibrocartilaginous discs that separate the bony surfaces
- Have a central *nucleus pulposus* of discs that cushions bony contact

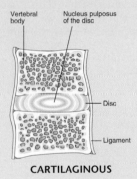

CARTILAGINOUS

Fibrous Joints

- No appreciable movement
- Consist of fibrous tissue or cartilage
- Lack a joint cavity

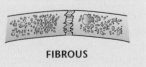

FIBROUS

Review the types of synovial joints and their associated features as well.

THE HEALTH HISTORY

Begin with "Any pains in your back?" because *backache* is the most common and widespread disorder of the musculoskeletal system. Establish whether the pain is on midline, in the area of the vertebrae, or off midline. If the pain radiates into the legs, ask about any associated numbness, tingling, or weakness.

See Table 15-1, Low Back Pain, pp. 255–256. Causes of midline back pain include musculoskeletal strain, vertebral collapse, disc herniation, or spinal cord metastases. Pain off the midline may arise from sacroiliitis, trochanteric bursitis, sciatica, or arthritis in the hips.

Proceed with "Do you have any pains in your joints?" If yes, you will need to determine whether the pain is *localized* or *widespread, acute* or *chronic, inflammatory* or *noninflammatory.*

Ask the patient to *point to the pain.* If the joint pain is localized and involves only one joint, it is *monoarticular.*

Pain in one joint suggests trauma, monoarticular arthritis, possible tendonitis, or bursitis. Hip pain near the greater trochanter suggests *trochanteric bursitis.*

If *polyarticular,* what is the pattern of involvement . . . migrating from joint to joint or steadily spreading from one joint to multiple joint involvement? Is the involvement symmetric?

Joint pain may be *nonarticular,* involving bones, muscles, and tissues around the joint such as the tendons, bursae, or even overlying skin. Generalized "aches and pains" are called *myalgias* if in muscles and *arthralgias* if in joints with no evidence of arthritis.

Problems in tissues around joints include inflammation of bursae (*bursitis*), tendons (*tendonitis*), or tendon sheaths (*tenosynovitis*); also *sprains* from stretching or tearing of ligaments

Assess the timing, quality, and severity of joint symptoms. *Timing* is especially important. If the pain comes from trauma, what was the *mechanisms of injury* or the series of events that caused the joint pain? Further, what aggravates or relieves the pain? What are the effects of exercise, rest, and treatment?

Severe pain of rapid onset in a swollen joint in the absence of trauma seen in acute septic arthritis or gout.

Determine if the problem is *inflammatory* or *noninflammatory.* Is there *tenderness, warmth,* or *redness?*

Fever, chills, warmth, redness in septic arthritis; also consider gout or rheumatic fever

Is the pain *articular* in origin, with *swelling, stiffness,* or *decreased range of motion?*

Pain, swelling, loss of active and passive motion, "locking," deformity in *articular joint pain;* loss of active but not passive motion, tenderness outside the joint, no deformity in *nonarticular pain*

Assess any *limitations of motion.*

Ask about any *systemic* features such as fever, chills, rash, anorexia, weight loss, and weakness.

Generalized symptoms are common in rheumatoid arthritis, *systemic lupus erythematosus, polymyalgia rheumatica*, and other inflammatory arthritides. High fever and chills suggest an infectious cause.

HEALTH PROMOTION AND COUNSELING

Important Topics for Health Promotion and Counseling

- Balanced nutrition, exercise, appropriate weight
- Lifting and the biomechanics of the back
- Risk-factor screening and prevention of falls
- Counseling about prevention and treatment of osteoporosis

A healthy lifestyle conveys direct benefits to the skeleton. Counsel patients that good nutrition supplies calcium needed for bone mineralization and bone density. Exercise appears to maintain and possibly increase bone mass, in addition to improving outlook and stress management. Weight appropriate to height and body frame reduces excess mechanical wear on weight-bearing joints such as hips and knees.

One of the most vulnerable parts of the skeleton is the low back, especially L5–S1, where the sacral vertebrae make a sharp posterior angle. More than 80% of the population experiences low back pain at least once. Exercises to strengthen the low back, especially in flexion and extension, and general fitness exercises appear equally effective. Education on lifting strategies, posture, and the biomechanics of injury is prudent for nurses, heavy-machinery operators, and construction workers.

Among older adults in the United States, falls are the leading cause of nonfatal injuries and account for a dramatic rise in death rates after 65 years of age. Risk factors are both cognitive and physiologic, including unstable gait, imbalanced posture, reduced strength, cognitive loss as in dementia, deficits in vision and proprioception, and osteoporosis. Urge patients to correct poor lighting, stairs, and chairs at awkward heights, slippery or irregular surfaces, and ill-fitting shoes. Scrutinize any medications affecting balance, especially benzodiazepines, vasodilators, and diuretics.

Counsel selected postmenopausal women about hormone replacement therapy and osteoporosis, defined as bone density >2.5 standard deviations below normal bone mass in young women. A 10% drop in bone mineral density, equivalent to one standard deviation, is associated with a 20% increase in risk of fracture. At highest risk are women of Caucasian origin or slender build, or with prior history of bilateral oophorectomy before menopause.

Criteria are unclear for identifying those women at menopause at greatest risk of bone loss and fractures 1 to 2 decades later. In addition, guidelines for tailoring dosage of medication to level of bone density have yet to be determined. Several agents inhibit bone resorption—calcium, vitamin D, calcitonin, bisphosphonates, and estrogen. Estrogen therapy appears most beneficial when started near menopause; however, recommendations about its risks and benefits continue to fluctuate.

TECHNIQUES OF EXAMINATION

General Approach

Inspect the joints and surrounding tissues as you examine the various body parts.

Identify joints with changes in structure and function, carefully assessing for:

- Symmetry of involvement—one or both sides of the body; one joint or several

- Deformity or malalignment of bones

- Changes in surrounding soft tissue—skin changes, subcutaneous nodules, muscle atrophy, crepitus

- Limitations in range of motion, ligamentous laxity

- Changes in muscle strength

Note signs of inflammation and arthritis: swelling, warmth, tenderness, redness.

TECHNIQUES	POSSIBLE FINDINGS

TEMPOROMANDIBULAR JOINT

Palpate the temporomandibular joint as the patient opens and closes the mouth.

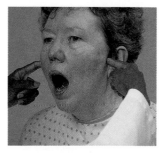

TECHNIQUES	**POSSIBLE FINDINGS**

SHOULDERS

Inspect the contour of the shoulders and shoulder girdles from front and back.

Muscle atrophy; anterior or posterior dislocation of humeral head

Ask patient to:

- Raise the arms to shoulder level, palms facing down.

Impaired glenohumeral motion

- Raise the arms vertically above the head, palms facing each other.

Impaired scapulothoracic motion (first 60°), impaired scapulothoracic and glenohumeral motion (final 30°)

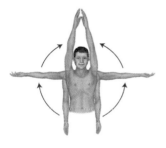

- Place both hands behind the neck, with elbows out (abduction and external rotation).

Impaired *external rotation* of shoulder, as in arthritis, bursitis

- Place both hands behind the small of the back (adduction and internal rotation).

Impaired *internal rotation* of shoulder, as in arthritis, bursitis

Assess areas of pain or tenderness.

TECHNIQUES	**POSSIBLE FINDINGS**
■ *Acromioclavicular joint:* palpate; adduct arm across chest (crossover test).	Arthritis, inflammation
■ *Subacromial and subdeltoid bursa:* lift elbow posteriorly; palpate anterior to acromion and over subdeltoid bursa.	Subacromial or subdeltoid bursitis

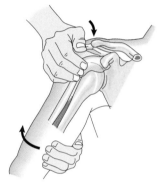

■ *Rotator cuff:* lift elbow posteriorly; palpate head of humerus for tenderness over tendon insertions of "SITS" muscles (supraspinatus, infraspinatus, teres minor; subscapularis not palpable).	Rotator cuff tendonitis

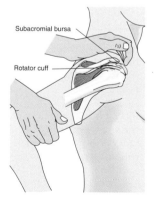

TECHNIQUES	**POSSIBLE FINDINGS**

Check for ability to raise arm to shoulder level ("drop-arm" sign).

Inability to raise or maintain arm at shoulder level indicates *rotator cuff sprain or tear.*

■ *Bicipital groove and tendon:* rotate humerus externally; palpate bicipital groove: alternately, with forearm flexed at right angle, supinate forearm against resistance.

Bicipital tenderness

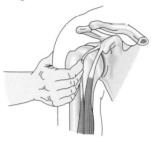

ELBOWS

Inspect and **palpate**

■ Olecranon process

Olecranon bursitis; posterior dislocation from direct trauma or supracondylar fracture

■ Medial and lateral epicondyles

Tender in epicondylitis

■ Extensor surface of the ulna

Rheumatoid nodules

■ Grooves overlying the elbow joint

Tender in arthritis

Ask patient to

■ Flex and extend elbows

■ Turn palms up and down (supination and pronation)

TECHNIQUES	POSSIBLE FINDINGS

WRISTS AND HANDS

Inspect

■ Movement of the wrist (flexion, extension, ulnar and medial deviation), hands, and fingers

Guarded movement in injury

■ Contours of wrists, hands, fingers

Deformities in rheumatoid and degenerative arthritis; swelling in arthritis, ganglia; impaired alignment of fingers in flexor tendon damage

■ Contours in palms

Thenar atrophy in median nerve compression (carpal tunnel syndrome); hypothenar atrophy in ulnar nerve compression

Palpate

■ Wrist joints

Swelling in rheumatoid arthritis, gonococcal infection of joint or extensor tendon sheaths

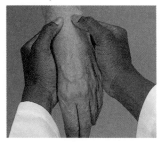

■ Distal radius and ulna

Tenderness over ulnar styloid in Colles' fracture

TECHNIQUES	POSSIBLE FINDINGS

■ "Anatomic snuffbox," the hollow space distal to the radial styloid bone

Tenderness suggests scaphoid fracture.

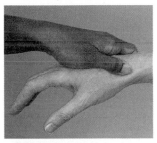

■ Metacarpophalangeal joint

Swelling in rheumatoid arthritis

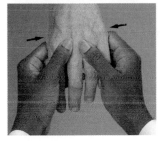

■ Proximal and distal interphalangeal joint

Proximal nodules in rheumatoid arthritis (Bouchard's nodes), distal nodules in osteoarthritis (Heberden's nodes)

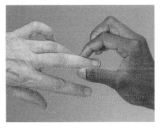

TECHNIQUES	**POSSIBLE FINDINGS**

SPINE

Inspect spine from side and back, noting any abnormal curvatures.

Kyphosis, scoliosis, lordosis, gibbus, list curvatures

Look for asymmetries of shoulders, iliac crests, or buttocks.

Pelvic tilt

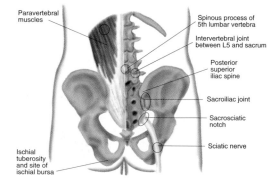

Paraverbral muscles

Spinous process of 5th lumbar vertebra

Intervertebral joint between L5 and sacrum

Posterior superior iliac spine

Sacroiliac joint

Sacrosciatic notch

Sciatic nerve

Ischial tuberosity and site of ischial bursa

Identify and **palpate**

- Spinous processes of each vertebra

Tender if trauma, infection

"Step offs" in spondylolisthesis, fracture

- Sacroiliac joint

Sacroiliitis

- Paravertebral muscles, if painful

Paravertebral muscle spasm in abnormal posture, degenerative and inflammatory muscle processes

TECHNIQUES	**POSSIBLE FINDINGS**

■ Sciatic nerve (midway between greater trochanter and ischial tuberosity)

Herniated disc nerve root compression

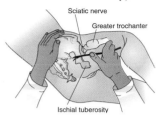

Test the range of motion in the neck and spine in

Decreased mobility in arthritis

■ Flexion

■ Extension

■ Rotation

■ Lateral bending

HIPS

Inspect gait for

■ Stance (see below) and swing (foot moves forward, does not bear weight)

Most problems appear during weight-bearing stance phase.

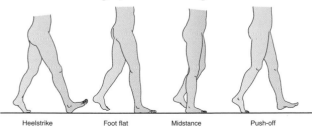

| Heelstrike | Foot flat | Midstance | Push-off |

THE STANCE PHASE OF GAIT

TECHNIQUES	POSSIBLE FINDINGS
■ Width of base (usually 2 to 4 inches from heel to heel) shift of pelvis, flexion of knee	Cerebellar disease or foot problems in wide base; impaired shift of pelvis in arthritis, hip dislocation, abductor weakness; disrupted gain in lack of knee flexion

Palpate

■ Along the inguinal ligament	Bulges in inguinal hernia, aneurysm
■ The *iliopectineal bursa*, lateral to the femoral pulse	Tender in synovitis, bursitis, iliopsoas abscess
■ The *trochanteric bursa*, on the greater trochanter of the femur	Tender in trochanteric bursitis
■ The *ischiogluteal bursa*, superficial to the ischial tuberosity	Tender in bursitis ("weaver's bottom")

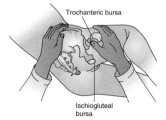

Trochanteric bursa

Ischiogluteal bursa

TROCHANTERIC BURSA

Check range of motion including

■ Flexion	Flexion of opposite leg suggests deformity of that hip.

TECHNIQUES	**POSSIBLE FINDINGS**

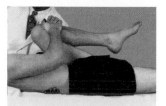

**HIP FLEXION AND
FLATTENING OF
LUMBAR LORDOSIS**

■ Extension   Painful in iliopsoas abscess

■ Abduction   Restricted in arthritis

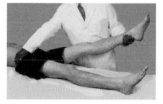

■ Adduction

■ Internal and external   Restricted in arthritis
   rotation

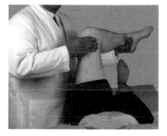

TECHNIQUES	POSSIBLE FINDINGS

KNEES

Review the structures of the knee.

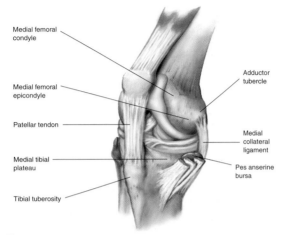

Medial femoral condyle

Medial femoral epicondyle

Patellar tendon

Medial tibial plateau

Tibial tuberosity

Adductor tubercle

Medial collateral ligament

Pes anserine bursa

Inspect

■ Gait for knee extension at heel strike, flexion during all other phases of swing and stance	Stumbling or pushing knee into extension in quadriceps weakness
■ Alignment of knees	Bowlegs, knock-knees; flexion contractures in limb paralysis
■ Contours of knees including any atrophy of the quadriceps muscles	Quadriceps atrophy with patellofemoral disorder

Inspect and palpate

■ Patella	Swelling of prepatellar bursitis ("housemaid's knee"), if over the patella

TECHNIQUES	POSSIBLE FINDINGS
■ Suprapatellar pouch	Swelling in synovitis and arthritis
■ Infrapatellar spaces (hollow areas adjacent to patella)	Swelling in arthritis
■ Medial tibial condyle	Swelling in *pes anserine* bursitis
■ Popliteal surface	Popliteal or "Baker's" cyst
Assess the patellofemoral compartment.	
■ Palpate the patellar tendon and ask patient to extend the leg.	Tenderness or inability to extend the leg in partial or complete tear of the patellar tendon
■ Press the patella against the underlying femur.	Pain, crepitus, and a history of knee pain suggest a patellofemoral disorder.
■ Push patella distally and ask patient to tighten knee against table.	Pain during contraction of quadriceps suggests *chondromalacia*.
With knees flexed, **palpate**	
■ Medial and lateral menisci	Tenderness in medial or lateral meniscus tear
■ Medial collateral ligaments (MCLs) and lateral collateral ligaments (LCLs)	Tenderness in MCL or LCL sprain
Assess any effusions.	

TECHNIQUES	POSSIBLE FINDINGS

- The *Bulge Sign* for minor effusions: Compress the suprapatellar pouch, stroke downward on medial surface, apply pressure to force fluid to lateral surface, then tap knee behind lateral margin of patella

A fluid wave returning to the medial surface after a lateral tap confirms an effusion—a positive "bulge sign."

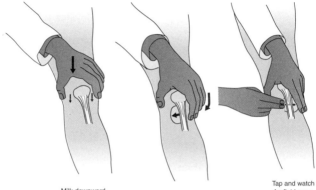

Milk downward

Apply medial pressure

Tap and watch for fluid wave

- The *Balloon Sign* for major effusions: Compress the suprapatellar pouch with one hand and with thumb and finger of the other, feel for fluid entering the spaces next to the patella.

A palpable fluid wave is a positive sign.

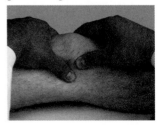

TECHNIQUES	**POSSIBLE FINDINGS**

■ *Ballotting the patella* for major effusions: Push the patella sharply against the femur; watch for fluid returning to the suprapatellar space.

Visible wave is a positive sign.

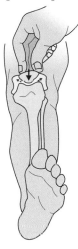

If painful, **assess** ligaments.

■ *Medial collateral ligament:* With knee slightly flexed, push medially against lateral surface of knee with one hand and pull laterally at the ankle with the other hand (an *abduction* or *valgus stress*).

Pain or a gap in the medial joint line points to a partial or complete MCL tear.

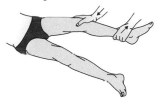

TECHNIQUES	POSSIBLE FINDINGS

■ *Lateral collateral ligament:* With knee slightly flexed, push laterally along medial surface of knee with one hand and pull medially at the ankle with the other hand (an *adduction* or *varus stress*).

Pain or a gap in the lateral joint line points to a partial or complete LCL tear (less common than MCL injuries).

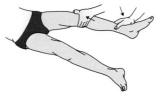

■ *Anterior cruciate ligament (ACL):* With knee flexed, place thumbs on medial and lateral joint line and place fingers on hamstring insertions. Pull tibia forward and observe if it slides forward "like a drawer." Compare the degree of forward movement to that of the opposite knee.

If the proximal tibia slides forward, there is a positive *anterior drawer sign,* suggesting ACL ligamentous laxity or an ACL tear.

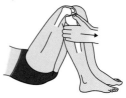

■ Apply the *Lachman test:* Grasp the distal femur with one hand and the proximal tibia with the other (place the thumb on the joint line). Move the femur forward and the tibia back.

Significant forward excursion of the tibia suggests ACL tear.

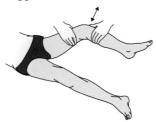

TECHNIQUES	**POSSIBLE FINDINGS**

- *Posterior cruciate ligament (PCL):* Position the patient and examining hands as described in the ACL test. Push the tibia posteriorly and observe for posterior movement.

Isolated PCL tears are rare.

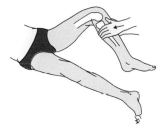

- *Medial meniscus and lateral meniscus:* With the patient supine, grasp the heel and flex the knee. Cup your other hand over the knee joint with fingers and thumb along the medial and lateral joint line. From the heel, rotate the lower leg internally and externally. Then push on the lateral side to apply a valgus stress on the medial side of the joint. At the same time, rotate the leg externally and slowly extend it.

A click or pop along the medial joint with valgus stress, external rotation, and leg extension suggests a probable tear of the posterior portion of the medial meniscus.

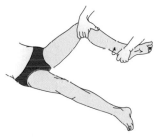

ANKLES AND FEET

Inspect ankles and feet.	Hallux valgus, corns, calluses
Palpate	
■ Ankle joint and ligaments	Tender joint in arthritis, tender ligaments in sprain

TECHNIQUES	**POSSIBLE FINDINGS**

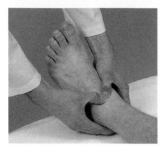

- Achilles tendon

  Rheumatoid nodules, tenderness in tendonitis

- **Compress** the metatarsophalangeal joints; then **palpate** each joint between the thumb and forefinger.

  Tenderness in arthritis and other conditions

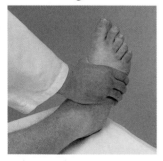 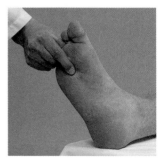

Assess range of motion.

- Dorsiflex and plantar flex the ankle (*tibiotalar joint*).

  An arthritic joint often hurts when moved in any direction. A sprain hurts chiefly when the injured ligament is stretched.

TECHNIQUES	POSSIBLE FINDINGS

■ Stabilize the ankle and invert and evert the heel (*subtalar* or *talocalcaneal joint*).

Ankle sprain

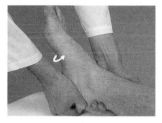

INVERSION

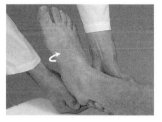

EVERSION

■ Stabilize the heel and invert and evert the forefoot (*transverse tarsal joints*).

Trauma, arthritis

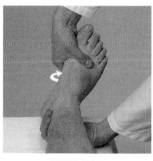

INVERSION

EVERSION

■ Flex toes at metatarsophalangeal joints.

TECHNIQUES	POSSIBLE FINDINGS

SPECIAL TECHNIQUE

Carpal Tunnel Syndrome.
Appropriate symptoms and objective loss of sensation on the ventral surface of the hand in the distribution of the median nerve and *weak abduction of the thumb* on muscle strength testing are the most helpful for making the diagnosis. Tinel's test appears more likely than Phalen's test to be confirmed by further diagnostic testing.

Thumb Adduction. Ask patient to raise the thumb perpendicular to the palm as you apply downward pressure on the distal phalanx. (This maneuver reliably tests the strength of the abductor pollicis brevis, which is innervated only by the median nerve.)

Tinel's Sign. Percuss lightly over median nerve at wrist.

Tingling or electric sensations in the distribution of the median nerve constitute a *positive* sign.

Phalen's Test. Hold patient's wrists in acute flexion, or ask patient to press backs of both hands together to form right angles. Either position should be held for 60 seconds.

Numbness or tingling over distribution of median nerve is a positive sign, suggesting carpal tunnel syndrome.

| **TECHNIQUES** | **POSSIBLE FINDINGS** |

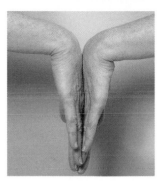

○— **Straight Leg Raising.** Raise patient's straightened leg until pain occurs. Then dorsiflex foot.

Sharp pain down back of leg suggests tension on or compression of a nerve root. Dorsiflexion increases pain.

○— **Measuring Leg Length.** Patient's legs should be aligned symmetrically. With a tape, measure distance from anterior superior iliac spine to medial malleolus. Tape should cross knee medially.

Unequal leg length may be the cause of scoliosis.

/○— **Measuring Range of Motion.** To measure range of motion precisely, a simple pocket goniometer is needed. Estimates may be made visually. Movement in the elbow at the right is limited to range indicated by red lines.

A flexion deformity of 45° and further flexion to 90° (45° → 90°).

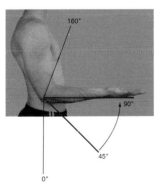

TECHNIQUES	POSSIBLE FINDINGS

Recording the Physical Examination— The Musculoskeletal System

"Good range of motion in all joints. No evidence of swelling or deformity."

OR

"Good range of motion in all joints. Hand with degenerative changes of Heberden's nodes at the distal interphalangeal joints, Bouchard's nodes at proximal interphalangeal joints. Mild pain with flexion, extension, and rotation of both hips. Good range of motion in the knees, with moderate crepitus; no effusion but boggy synovium and osteophytes along the tibiofemoral joint line bilaterally. Both feet with hallux valgus at the first metatarsophalangeal joints."

Suggests osteoarthritis

AIDS TO INTERPRETATION

TABLE 15-1 ■ Low Back Pain

Patterns	Physical Signs
Mechanical Low Back Pain	
Acute, often recurrent, or possibly chronic aching pain in the lumbrosacral area, possibly radiating into the posterior thighs but not below the knees. Often aggravated by moving, lifting, or twisting motions and relieved by rest. Spinal movements typically limited by pain. Cause unclear.	Local tenderness, muscle spasm, pain on movement of the back; loss of the normal lumbar lordosis but no motor or sensory loss or reflex abnormalities. In osteoporosis: possible thoracic kyphosis, percussion tenderness over a spinous process, or fractures elsewhere such as in the thoracic spine or in a hip.
Radicular Low Back Pain	
Radicular (nerve root) pain, usually superimposed on low back pain. Pain is shooting, radiates down one or both legs, usually to below the knee(s) in a dermatomal distribution, often with numbness, tingling, and local weakness. Pain often is worsened by spinal movement such as bending and by sneezing, coughing, or straining.	Pain on straight-leg raising, tenderness of the sciatic nerve, loss of sensation in a dermatomal distribution, local muscular weakness and atrophy, and decreased to absent reflex(es), especially affecting the ankle jerks. Dermatomal signs and reflex changes may be absent when only a single root is affected.
A herniated intervertebral disc with compression or traction of nerve root(s) in persons younger than 50, usually affecting nerve roots of L5 or S1. Spinal cord tumors, abscesses, much less common causes.	

(table continues next page)

TABLE 15-1 ■ Low Back Pain *(Continued)*	
Patterns	**Physical Signs**
Back and Leg Pain From Lumbar Stenosis	
Pseudoclaudication is pain in the back or legs that worsens with walking and improves with flexing of the spine, as by sitting or bending forward.	Lumbar stenosis, a combination of degenerative disc disease and osteoarthritis that narrows the spinal canal and impinges on the spinal nerves. The posture may become flexed forward. Possible motor weakness and hyporeflexia in the lower extremities.
Chronic Persistent Low Back Stiffness	
Ankylosing spondylitis, a chronic inflammatory polyarthritis, most common in young men; diffuse idiopathic skeletal hyperostosis (DISH), which affects middle-aged and older men	Loss of the normal lumbar lordosis, muscle spasm, and limitation of anterior and lateral flexion; flexion and immobility of the spine
Aching Nocturnal Back Pain, Unrelieved by Rest	
Consider metastatic malignancy in the spine, as from cancer of the prostate, breast, lung, thyroid, and kidney, and multiple myeloma.	Findings vary with the source. Local bone tenderness may be present.
Back Pain Referred From the Abdomen or Pelvis	
Usually a deep, aching pain, the level of which varies with the source	Spinal movements are not painful and range of motion is not affected. Look for signs of the primary disorder.

TABLE 15-2 ■ Patterns of Pain in and Around the Joints		
	Rheumatoid Arthritis	**Osteoarthritis (Degenerative Joint Disease or DJD)**
Process	Chronic inflammation of synovial membranes with secondary erosion of adjacent cartilage and bone, and damage to ligaments and tendons	Degeneration and progressive loss of cartilage within the joints, damage to underlying bone, and formation of new bone at the margins of the cartilage
Common Locations	Hands (proximal interphalangeal and metacarpophalangeal joints), feet (metatarsophalangeal joints), wrists, knees, elbows, ankles	Knees, hips, hands (distal, sometimes proximal interphalangeal joints), cervical and lumbar spine, and wrists (first carpometacarpal joint); also joints previously injured or diseased
Pattern of Spread	Symmetrically additive: progresses to other joints while persisting in the initial ones	Additive; however, only one joint may be involved
Onset	Usually insidious	Usually insidious
Progression and Duration	Often chronic, with remissions and exacerbations	Slowly progressive, with temporary exacerbations after periods of overuse

(table continues next page)

TABLE 15-2 ■ Patterns of Pain in and Around the Joints *(Continued)*		
	Rheumatoid Arthritis	**Osteoarthritis (Degenerative Joint Disease or DJD)**
Associated Symptoms	Frequent swelling of synovial tissue in joints or tendon sheaths; also subcutaneous nodules	Small effusions in the joints may be present, especially in the knees; also bony enlargement.
	Tender, often warm, but seldom red	Possibly tender, seldom warm, and rarely red
	Prominent stiffness, often for 1 hour or more in the mornings, also after inactivity	Frequent but brief stiffness (usually 5–10 min), in the morning and after inactivity
	Limitation of motion common	Limitation of motion often develops
	Weakness, fatigue, weight loss, and low fever	

TABLE 15-3 ■ Painful Tender Shoulders

Acromioclavicular arthritis

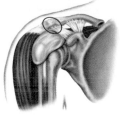

Tenderness over the acromioclavicular joint, especially with adduction of the arm across the chest. Pain often increases with shrugging the shoulders.

Subacromial and subdeltoid bursitis

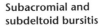
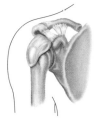

Pain over anterior superior aspect of shoulder, particularly when raising the arm overhead. Tenderness common anterolateral to the acromion, in hollow recess formed by the acromiohumeral sulcus. Often seen in overuse syndromes.

Rotator cuff tendinitis

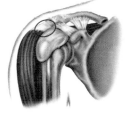

Tenderness over the rotator cuff, when elbow passively lifted posteriorly or with "drop arm" maneuver.

Bicipital tendinitis

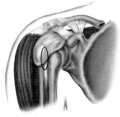

Tenderness over the long head of the biceps when rolled in the bicipital groove or when flexed arm is supinated against resistance suggests *bicipital tendinitis.*

TABLE 15-4 ■ Painful Tender Knees

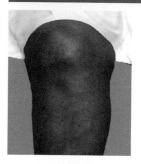

Arthritis. *Degenerative arthritis* usually occurs after age 50; associated with obesity. Often with medial joint line tenderness, palpable osteophytes, bowleg appearance, mild effusion. Systemic involvement, swelling, and subcutaneous nodules in *rheumatoid arthritis*.

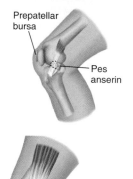

Prepatellar bursa

Pes anserin

Iliotibial band

Bursitis. Inflammation and thickening of bursa seen in repetitive motion and overuse syndromes. Can involve *prepatellar bursa* ("housemaid's knee"), *pes anserine* bursa medially (runners, osteoarthritis) *iliotibial band* laterally (over lateral femoral condyle), especially in runners.

(table continues next page)

TABLE 15-4 ■ Painful Tender Knees *(Continued)*

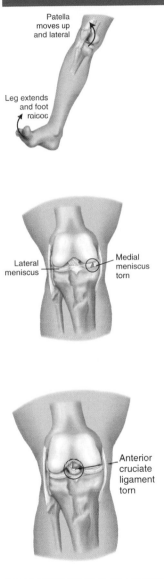

Patella moves up and lateral

Leg extends and foot raised

Lateral meniscus

Medial meniscus torn

Anterior cruciate ligament torn

Patellofemoral instability. During flexion and extension of knee, due to subluxation and/or malalignment. Patella tracks laterally instead of centrally in the trochlear groove of distal femoral condyle. Inspect or palpate for lateral motion with leg extension. May lead to chondromalacia or osteoarthritis.

Meniscal tear. Commonly arises from twisting injury of knee; in older patients may be degenerative. Patients report clicking, popping, or locking sensation. Check for tenderness along joint line over medial or lateral meniscus and for effusion. May be accompanied by associated tears of medial collateral or anterior cruciate ligaments.

Anterior cruciate tear or sprain. Also seen in twisting injuries of the knee. Patients report popping sensation, immediate swelling, pain with flexion and extension, difficulty walking, and eventually the sensation of the knee "giving way." Check for anterior drawer sign, swelling from hemarthrosis, and for
(table continues next page)

TABLE 15-4 ■ Painful Tender Knees *(Continued)*

associated injuries to medial meniscus or medial collateral ligament. Consider evaluation by orthopedic surgery.

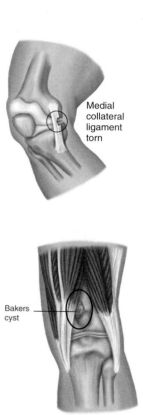

Medial collateral ligament torn

Posterior knee

POSTERIOR KNEE

Collateral ligament sprain or tear. Often arises from force applied to medial or lateral surface of knee (valgus or varus stress respectively), producing localized swelling, pain, and stiffness. Patients usually able to walk but may develop an effusion later. Physical findings include tenderness over the affected ligament and ligamentous laxity during valgus or varus stress.

Baker's cyst. Cystic swelling palpable on the medial surface of the popliteal fossa, prompting complaints of aching or fullness behind the knee. Inspect and palpate for cystic swelling adjacent to the medial hamstring tendons. Presence of an effusion suggests involvement of the posterior horn of the medial meniscus. In rheumatoid arthritis cyst may expand into calf or even the ankle.

Bakers cyst

The Nervous System

FUNDAMENTALS FOR ASSESSING THE NERVOUS SYSTEM

The *central nervous system* (CNS) consists of the brain and spinal cord. The *peripheral nervous system* consists of the 12 pairs of cranial nerves and the spinal and peripheral nerves. Most peripheral nerves contain both motor and sensory fibers.

■ Central Nervous System

THE BRAIN

- *Gray matter,* or aggregations of neuronal cell bodies; rims the surfaces of the cerebral hemispheres, forming the cerebral cortex

- *White matter,* or neuronal axons coated with myelin, allowing nerve impulses to travel more rapidly

- *Basal ganglia,* which affect movement

- *Thalamus,* which processes and relays sensory impulses to the cerebral cortex

- *Hypothalamus,* which maintains homeostasis and regulates temperature, heart rate, and blood pressure; affects endocrine system and governs emotional behaviors such as

anger and sex drive; and contains hormones that act
directly on the pituitary gland

- *Brainstem,* which connects the upper part of the brain
with the spinal cord and has three sections: midbrain,
pons, and medulla

- *Reticular activating (arousal) system,* in the diencephalon
and upper brainstem; activation linked to consciousness

- *Cerebellum,* at the base of the brain, which coordinates all
movement and helps maintain the body upright in space

THE SPINAL CORD

- A cylindrical mass of nerve tissue encased within the bony
vertebral column, extending from medulla to first or
second lumbar vertebra

- Contains important motor and sensory nerve pathways
that exit and enter the cord via anterior and posterior
nerve roots and spinal and peripheral nerves

- Mediates reflex activity of the deep tendon (or spinal
nerve) reflexes

- Divided into five segments: cervical (C1–8), thoracic
(T1–12), lumbar (L1–5), sacral (S1–5), and coccygeal

- Roots fan out like a horse's tail at L1–2, the *cauda equina*

Peripheral Nervous System

THE CRANIAL NERVES

- Cranial Nerves II through XII arise from the diencephalon
and brainstem.

- Cranial Nerves I and II are actually fiber tracts emerging
from the brain.

THE PERIPHERAL NERVES

■ Thirty-one pairs of nerves carry impulses to and from the cord: 8 cervical, 12 thoracic, 5 lumbar, 5 sacral, and 1 coccygeal.

■ Each nerve has an anterior (ventral) root containing motor fibers, and a posterior (dorsal) root containing sensory fibers.

■ These merge to form a short (<5 mm) *spinal nerve*.

■ Spinal nerve fibers commingle with similar fibers from other levels to form *peripheral nerves*.

THE HEALTH HISTORY

Common or Concerning Symptoms

■ Changes in mood, attention, or speech
■ Changes in orientation, memory, insight, or judgment
■ Delirium or dementia
■ Headache
■ Dizziness or vertigo
■ Generalized, proximal, or distal weakness
■ Numbness, abnormal or lost sensations
■ Loss of consciousness, syncope, or near-syncope
■ Seizures
■ Tremors or involuntary movements

Assess *level of consciousness*, general *appearance* and *mood*, and *ability to pay attention, remember, understand*, and *speak*. Assess patient's responses to illness and life circumstances, which often tell you about his or her *insight* and

See Table 16-1, Disorders of Speech, p. 294.

judgment. Test *orientation* and *memory.*

For *headache,* ask about location, severity, duration, and any associated symptoms, such as visual changes, weakness, or loss of sensation. Ask if coughing, sneezing, or sudden movements of the head affect the headache.

See Table 5-1, Headaches, pp. 84–88. *Subarachnoid hemorrhage* may evoke "the worst headache of my life." Dull headache affected by maneuvers, especially on awakening and in the same location, occurs with mass lesions such as brain tumors.

Dizziness can have many meanings. Is the patient lightheaded or feeling faint? Or is there *vertigo,* a perception that the room is spinning or rotating?

Lightheadedness in palpitations; near-syncope from vasovagal stimulation, low blood pressure, febrile illness, and others; vertigo in middle-ear conditions, brainstem tumor

Especially in older adults, are any medications contributing to dizziness? Are any associated symptoms present, such as double vision (*diplopia*), difficulty forming words (*dysarthria*), or difficulty with gait or balance (*ataxia*)?

Diplopia, dysarthria, ataxia in posterior circulation transient ischemic attack (TIA) or stroke

What about any associated *weakness?*

Weakness or paralysis in TIA or stroke

Try to distinguish between *proximal* and *distal weakness.* For proximal weakness, ask about combing hair, reaching for things on a high shelf, or difficulty getting out of a chair or taking a high step up. For

Bilateral proximal weakness in myopathy; bilateral, predominantly distal weakness in polyneuropathy; weakness worsened by repeated effort and improved by rest in myasthenia gravis distal weakness in the arms, inquire about hand movements such as opening a jar or can or using hand tools (e.g., scissors, pliers, screwdriver). For distal weakness in the legs, ask about frequent tripping.

Is there any *loss of sensation,* difficulty moving a limb, or altered sensations such as tingling or pins and needles? Peculiar sensations without an obvious stimulus (*paresthesias*)? *Dysesthesias,* or disordered sensations in response to a stimulus, may last longer than the stimulus itself.

Loss of sensation, paresthesias, and dysesthesias in central lesions of the brain and spinal cord, as well as in disorders of peripheral sensory roots and nerves; paresthesias in hands and around mouth in hyperventilation

"Have you ever fainted or passed out?" leads the discussion to any *loss of consciousness. Syncope* is the sudden but temporary loss of consciousness that occurs with decreased blood flow to the brain, commonly described as *fainting.*

Get as complete and unbiased a description of the event as you can. What brought on the episode? Were there any warning symptoms? Was the patient standing, sitting, or lying down when it began? How long did it last? Could voices be heard while passing out and coming to? How rapid

Young people with emotional stress and warning symptoms of flushing, warmth, or nausea may have *vasodepressor (or vasovagal) syncope* of slow onset, slow offset. *Cardiac syncope* from dysrhythmias, more common in older patients, often with sudden onset, sudden offset.

was recovery? In retrospect, were onset and offset slow or fast?

Also ask if anyone observed the episode. If so, what did the patient look like before losing consciousness, during the episode, and after? Was there any seizure-like movement of the arms or legs? Any incontinence of the bladder or bowel?

A *seizure* is a paroxysmal disorder caused by sudden excessive electrical discharge in the cerebral cortex or its underlying structures. Seizures can be of several types. Depending on the type, there may or may not be loss of consciousness. There may be abnormal feelings, thought processes, and sensations, including smells, as well as abnormal movements.

Tonic–clonic motor activity, incontinence, and *postictal state* suggest a generalized *seizure*. Unlike syncope, injury such as tongue biting or bruising of limbs may occur.

HEALTH PROMOTION AND COUNSELING

Important Topics for Health Promotion and Counseling

- Screening for depression and suicidality
- Screening for dementia
- Prevention of stroke

Lifetime prevalence of major depression meeting formal diagnostic criteria is 5% to 10% in men and 10% to 20% in women. Primary-care providers fail to diagnose major depression in up to 50% of affected patients, often missing early clues such as *low self-esteem, anhedonia* (lack of pleasure in daily activities), *sleep disorders,* and *difficulty concentrating* or *making decisions.* Failure to diagnose depression can have fatal consequences—suicide rates in patients with major depression are eight times higher than in the general population.*

Suicide rates are highest among men older than 65 years but have been increasing in teenagers and young adults. Risk factors include any history of psychiatric illness (especially linked to a hospital admission), substance abuse, personality disorder, prior suicide attempt, or family history of suicide. Clinicians should ask about domestic firearms and screen for alcohol dependence: guns are in the homes of more than 50% of all suicide victims, and alcohol intoxication is associated with nearly 25% of suicides. Any evidence of suicidal ideation must be further assessed.

Dementia, a "global impairment of cognitive function that interferes with normal activities,"** affects 16% of Americans older than 65 years. Most dementias represent Alzheimer's disease (~50%–85%) or vascular multi-infarct dementia (~10%–20%). Be watchful for Alzheimer's disease in people with a positive family history, because their risk is three times higher than in the general population.

Use of the Mini-Mental State Examination is helpful. Once cognitive change is identified, be sure to address the possible role of medications, depression, or metabolic abnormalities.

Incidence of stroke increases with age and is 60% higher in African Americans than in Caucasians. Control hypertension, which accelerates atherosclerotic changes in the carotid, vertebral, and cerebral arteries and disturbs autoregulation of cerebral blood pressure. Counsel patients to modify

*U.S. Preventive Services Task Force: Ch. 49: "Screening for Depression." In *Guide to Clinical Preventive Services.* Baltimore, Williams and Wilkins, pp. 541–546, 1996.
**U.S. Preventive Services Task Force: Ch. 48: "Screening for Dementia." In *Guide to Clinical Preventive Services.* Baltimore, Williams and Wilkins, pp. 531–541, 1996.

conditions contributing to atherosclerosis: smoking, hyperlipidemia, and diabetes. Warn drug users of the link between stroke and cocaine.

TECHNIQUES OF EXAMINATION

Three important questions govern the neurologic examination:

■ Is mental status intact?

■ Are right-sided and left-sided findings symmetric?

■ If findings are asymmetric or otherwise abnormal, does the causative lesion lie in the CNS or the peripheral nervous system?

TECHNIQUES	POSSIBLE FINDINGS

MENTAL STATUS

Observe patient's mental status throughout your interaction. **Test** specific functions if indicated during the interview or physical examination.

APPEARANCE AND BEHAVIOR

Assess the following:

Level of Consciousness.
Observe alertness and response to verbal and tactile stimuli.

Normal consciousness, lethargy, obtundation, stupor, coma (see pp. 304–305)

Posture and Motor Behavior.
Observe pace, range, character, and appropriateness of movements.

Restlessness, agitation, bizarre postures, immobility, involuntary movements

TECHNIQUES	POSSIBLE FINDINGS
Dress, Grooming, and Personal Hygiene	Fastidiousness, neglect
Facial Expressions. **Assess** during rest and interaction.	Anxiety, depression, elation, anger, responses to imaginary people or objects, withdrawal
Manner, Affect, and Relation to People and Things	

SPEECH AND LANGUAGE

Note quantity, rate, loudness, clarity, and fluency of speech. If indicated, test for aphasia.	Aphasia, dysphonia, dysarthria, changes with mood disorders

Testing for Aphasia	
Word Comprehension	Ask patient to follow a one-stage command, such as "Point to your nose." Try a two-stage command: "Point to your mouth, then your knee."
Repetition	Ask patient to repeat a phrase of one-syllable words (the most difficult repetition task): "No ifs, ands, or buts."
Naming	Ask patient to name the parts of a watch.
Reading Comprehension	Ask patient to read a paragraph aloud.
Writing	Ask patient to write a sentence.

TECHNIQUES	POSSIBLE FINDINGS

MOOD

Ask about patient's spirits. **Note** nature, intensity, duration, and stability of any abnormal mood. If indicated, **assess** risk of suicide.

Happiness, elation, depression, anxiety, anger, indifference

THOUGHT AND PERCEPTIONS

Thought Processes. **Assess** logic, relevance, organization, and coherence.

Derailments, flight of ideas, incoherence, confabulation, blocking

Thought Content. **Ask** about and explore any unusual or unpleasant thoughts.

Obsessions, compulsions, delusions, feelings of unreality

Perceptions. **Ask** about any unusual perceptions (e.g., seeing or hearing things).

Illusions, hallucinations

Insight and Judgment. **Assess** patient's insight into the illness and level of judgment used in making decisions or plans.

Recognition or denial of mental cause of symptoms; bizarre, impulsive, or unrealistic judgment

COGNITIVE FUNCTIONS

If indicated, **assess:**

Orientation to time, place, and person

Disorientation

Attention

■ *Digit span*—ability to repeat a series of numbers forward and then backward

Poor performance of digit span, serial 7s, and spelling backward is common in dementia and delirium but has other causes, too.

TECHNIQUES	POSSIBLE FINDINGS

- *Serial 7s*—ability to subtract 7 repeatedly, starting with 100

- *Spelling backward* of a five-letter word, such as W-O-R-L-D

Remote Memory (e.g., birthdays, anniversaries, social security number, schools, jobs, wars)

Impaired in late stages of dementia

Recent Memory (e.g., events of the day)

Recent memory and new learning ability impaired in dementia, delirium, and amnestic disorders

New Learning Ability— ability to repeat three or four words after a few minutes of unrelated activity

HIGHER COGNITIVE FUNCTIONS

If indicated, **assess:**

Information and Vocabulary. **Note** range and depth of patient's information, complexity of ideas expressed, and vocabulary used. For the fund of information, you also may ask names of presidents, other political figures, or large cities.

These attributes reflect intelligence, education, and cultural background. They are limited by mental retardation but are fairly well preserved in early dementia.

Calculating Abilities, such as addition, subtraction, and multiplication

Poor calculation in mental retardation and dementia

TECHNIQUES	POSSIBLE FINDINGS
Abstract Thinking—ability to respond abstractly to questions about ■ The meaning of *proverbs,* such as "A stitch in time saves nine" ■ The *similarities* of beings or things, such as a cat and a mouse or a piano and a violin	Concrete responses (observable details rather than concepts) are common in mental retardation, dementia, and delirium. Responses are sometimes bizarre in schizophrenia.
Constructional Ability. **Ask** patient ■ To copy figures such as circle, cross, diamond, and box, and two intersecting pentagons, or ■ To draw a clock face with numbers and hands	Impaired ability common in dementia and with parietal lobe damage

CRANIAL NERVES

Cranial Nerves and Function			
No.	**Cranial Nerve**	**Function**
I	Olfactory	Sense of smell
II	Optic	Vision
III	Oculomotor	Pupillary constriction, opening the eye, and most extraocular movements
IV	Trochlear	Downward, inward movement of the eye
VI	Abducens	Lateral deviation of the eye
		(continued)

Cranial Nerves and Function (Continued)

No.	Cranial Nerve	Function
V	Trigeminal	*Motor*—temporal and masseter muscles (jaw clenching), also lateral movement of the jaw *Sensory*—facial. The nerve has three divisions: (1) ophthalmic, (2) maxillary, and (3) mandibular.
VII	Facial	*Motor*—facial movements, including those of facial expression, closing the eye, and closing the mouth *Sensory*—taste for salty, sweet, sour, and bitter substances on the anterior two thirds of the tongue
VIII	Acoustic	Hearing (cochlear division) and balance (vestibular division)
IX	Glossopharyngeal	*Motor*—pharynx *Sensory*—posterior portions of the eardrum and ear canal, the pharynx, and the posterior tongue, including taste (salty, sweet, sour, bitter)
X	Vagus	*Motor*—palate, pharynx, and larynx *Sensory*—pharynx and larynx
XI	Spinal accessory	*Motor*—the sternomastoid and upper portion of the trapezius
XII	Hypoglossal	*Motor*—tongue

CN I (OLFACTORY)

Test sense of smell on each side.　　　Loss in frontal lobe lesions

CN II (OPTIC)

Assess visual acuity.　　　Blindness

Check visual fields.　　　Hemianopsia

Inspect optic discs.　　　Papilledema, optic atrophy

TECHNIQUES	**POSSIBLE FINDINGS**

CN II, III (OPTIC AND OCULOMOTOR)

Test papillary reactions to light. If abnormal, test reactions to near effort.

Blindness, CN III paralysis, tonic pupils; Horner's syndrome may affect light reactions

CN III, IV, VI (OCULOMOTOR, TROCHLEAR, AND ABDUCENS)

Assess extraocular movements.

Strabismus from paralysis of CN III, IV, or VI; nystagmus

CN V (TRIGEMINAL)

Feel the contractions of temporal and masseter muscles.

Motor or sensory loss from lesions of CN V or its higher motor pathways

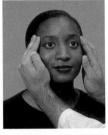

PALPATING TEMPORAL MUSCLES

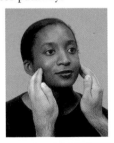

PALPATING MASSETER MUSCLES

Check corneal reflexes.

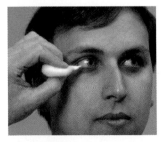

TECHNIQUES	POSSIBLE FINDINGS

Test pain and light touch sensations on face.

CN VII (FACIAL)

Ask patient to raise both eyebrows, frown, close eyes tightly, show teeth, smile, and puff out cheeks.

Weakness from lesion of peripheral nerve, as in Bell's palsy, or of CNS, as in a stroke. See Table 16-3, Facial Paralysis, p. 296.

CN VIII (ACOUSTIC)

Assess hearing. If decreased:

■ Test for lateralization (**Weber test**).

Sensorineural loss causes lateralization to less affected ear and AC > BC. Conduction loss causes lateralization to more affected ear and BC > AC.

■ Compare air and bone conduction (**Rinne test**).

CN IX, X (GLOSSOPHARYNGEAL AND VAGUS)

Observe any difficulty swallowing.

A weakened palate or pharynx impairs swallowing.

Listen to the voice.

Hoarseness or nasality

Watch soft palate rise with "ah."

Palatal paralysis

Test gag reflex on each side.

Absent reflex

CN XI (SPINAL ACCESSORY)

Trapezius Muscles. **Assess** muscles for bulk, involuntary movements, and strength of shoulder shrug.

Atrophy, fasciculations, weakness

TECHNIQUES	**POSSIBLE FINDINGS**

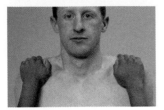

Sternomastoid Muscles.
Assess strength as head
turns against your hand.

Weakness

CN XII (HYPOGLOSSAL)

Listen to patient's
articulation.

Dysarthria from damage to
CN X or CN XII

Inspect the resting tongue.

Atrophy, fasciculations

Inspect the protruded
tongue.

Deviation to weak side

THE MOTOR SYSTEM

BODY POSITION

Observe the patient's body
position during movement
and at rest.

Hemiplegia in stroke

INVOLUNTARY MOVEMENTS

If present, **observe** location,
quality, rate, rhythm,
amplitude, and setting.

Tremors, fasciculations, tics,
chorea, athetosis, oral–facial
dyskinesias

MUSCLE BULK

Inspect muscle contours.

Atrophy

MUSCLE TONE

Assess resistance to passive
stretch of arms and legs.

Spasticity, rigidity, flaccidity

MUSCLE STRENGTH

Test and grade the major
muscle groups:

Grade	Description
Grading Muscle Strength	
0	No muscular contraction detected
1	A barely detectable trace of contraction
2	Active movement with gravity eliminated
3	Active movement against gravity
4	Active movement against gravity and some resistance
5	Active movement against full resistance

■ Elbow flexion (C5, C6)—
  biceps

■ Elbow extension (C6, C7,
  C8)—triceps

■ Wrist extension (C6, C7,
  C8, radial nerve)

■ Grip (C7, C8, T1)

■ Finger abduction
  (C8, T1)—ulnar nerve

Look for a pattern in any
detectable weakness. It may
suggest a lower motor
neuron lesion affecting a
peripheral nerve or nerve
root. Weakness of one side
of body suggests an upper
motor neuron lesion. A
polyneuropathy causes
symmetric distal weakness,
and a myopathy usually
causes proximal weakness.
Weakness that worsens with
repeated effort and improves
with rest suggests
myasthenia gravis.

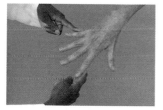

TECHNIQUES	**POSSIBLE FINDINGS**

■ Thumb opposition (C8, T1, median nerve)

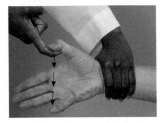

■ Trunk—flexion, extension, lateral bending

■ / Hip flexion (L2, L3, L4)—iliopsoas

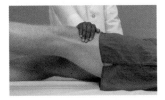

■ Hip adduction (L2, L3, L4)—adductors

■ Hip abduction (L4, L5, S1)—sulcus medius and minimus

■ Hip extension (S1)—gluteus maximus

■ Knee extension (L2, L3, L4)—quadriceps

■ Knee flexion (L4, L5, S1, S2)—hamstrings

TECHNIQUES	POSSIBLE FINDINGS

- Ankle dorsiflexion (L4, L5)

- Ankle plantar flexion (S1)

COORDINATION
Check:

Rapid alternating movements in arms and legs	Clumsy, slow movements in cerebellar disease
Point-to-point movements in arms and legs	Clumsy, unsteady movements in cerebellar disease

Gait. **Ask** patient to

■ Walk away, turn, and come back	Upper or lower motor neuron weakness, cerebellar ataxia, parkinsonism, and loss of position sense may all affect performance.

- Walk heel-to-toe

- Walk on toes, then on heels

- Hop in place on each foot

- Do one-legged shallow knee bends

(Substitute rising from a chair and climbing on a stool for hops and bends as indicated.)

TECHNIQUES	**POSSIBLE FINDINGS**

Stance

■ **Do** a *Romberg test* (a sensory test of stance). **Ask** patient to stand with feet together and eyes open, then closed for 20 to 30 seconds. Mild swaying may occur. (Stand close by to prevent falls.)

Loss of balance that appears when eyes are closed is a *positive* Romberg test, suggesting poor position sense.

■ Look for a *pronator drift*. Watch as patient holds arms forward, with eyes closed, for 20 to 30 seconds.

Flexion and pronation at elbow and downward drift of arm in hemiplegia

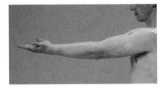

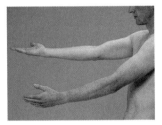

Ask patient to keep arms up and **tap** them downward. A smooth return to position is normal.

Weakness, incoordination, poor position sense

THE SENSORY SYSTEM

METHODS OF TESTING

⎞/○— **Compare** symmetric areas on the two sides of the body.

Hemisensory deficits

Also **compare** distal and proximal areas of arms and legs for *pain, temperature,*

"Glove-and-stocking" loss of peripheral neuropathy

TECHNIQUES	POSSIBLE FINDINGS

and *touch sensation*. Scatter stimuli to sample most dermatomes and major peripheral nerves.

Check fingers and toes distally for *vibration and position senses*. If responses are abnormal, test more proximally.

Loss of position and vibration senses in posterior column disease

Map any area of abnormal response, including dermatomes, if present.

Dermatomal sensory loss in *herpes zoster nerve root compression*

Assess response to the following stimuli (except when you are explaining the tests, patient's eyes should be closed):

■ *Pain.* Use the sharp end of a pin or other suitable tool. The dull end serves as a control.

Analgesia, hypalgesia, hyperalgesia

■ *Temperature* (if indicated). Use test tubes with hot and ice-cold water (or other objects of suitable temperature).

Temperature and pain senses usually correlate.

■ *Light touch.* Use a fine wisp of cotton.

Anesthesia, hyperesthesia

■ *Vibration.* Use a 128-Hz or 256-Hz tuning fork, held on a *bony* prominence.

Vibration and position senses, both carried in the posterior columns, often correlate.

TECHNIQUES	POSSIBLE FINDINGS

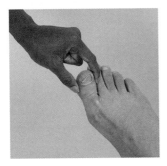

■ *Position.* Holding patient's finger or big toe by its sides, move it up or down.

Also assess one or more of the *discriminative* sensations:

■ *Stereognosis.* Ask for identification of a common object placed in patient's hand.

Lesions in the posterior columns or sensory cortex may impair stereognosis, number identification, and two-point discrimination.

■ *Number identification.*
Ask for identification of a
number drawn on
patient's palm with blunt
end of a pen.

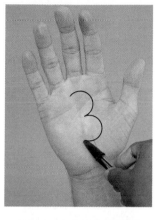

■ *Two-point discrimination.*
Find minimal distance on
pad of patient's finger at
which the sides of two
points can be distinguished
from one (normally
<5 mm).

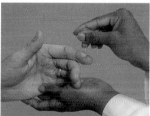

■ *Point localization.* Touch
skin briefly, and ask
patient to open both eyes
and identify the place
touched.

A lesion in the sensory
cortex may impair point
localization on the opposite
side and cause extinction of
the touch sensation on that
side.

■ *Extinction.*
Simultaneously touch
opposite, corresponding
areas of the body, and ask
patient where the touch
is felt.

TECHNIQUES	POSSIBLE FINDINGS

⌐o— *REFLEXES*

Grading Reflexes	
Grade	**Description**
4+	Hyperactive (with clonus)
3+	Brisker than average, not necessarily abnormal
2+	**Average, normal**
1+	Diminished, low normal
0	No response

Biceps (C5, C6)

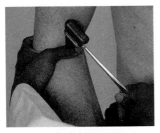

PATIENT SITTING

Triceps (C6, C7)

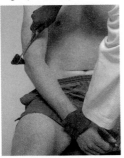

PATIENT SITTING

Hyperactive deep tendon reflexes, absent abdominal reflexes, and a Babinski response indicate an upper motor neuron lesion.

TECHNIQUES	POSSIBLE FINDINGS

Supinator (brachioradialis)
(C5, C6)

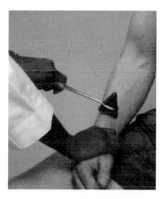

○— Abdominals (upper T8,
T9, T10; lower T10, T11,
T12)

May be absent with upper or
lower neuron lesions

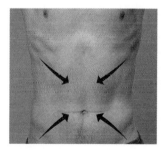

Upper (T8, T9, T10)

Lower (T10, T11, T12)

TECHNIQUES	POSSIBLE FINDINGS

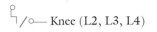
/o— Knee (L2, L3, L4)

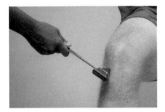

Ankle (S1)

Ankle jerks symmetrically decreased or absent in peripheral polyneuropathy

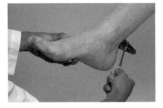

Plantar (L5, S1), normally flexor

Babinski response

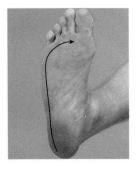

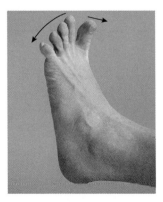

TECHNIQUES	POSSIBLE FINDINGS

Check for clonus if reflexes seem hyperactive.

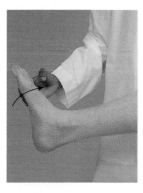

SPECIAL TECHNIQUE

Mini-Mental State Examination (MMSE). This brief test is useful in screening for cognitive dysfunction or dementia and following its course. For more detailed information, contact Publisher, Psychological Assessment Resources, Inc., 16204 North Florida Avenue, Lutz, FL 33549.

Asterixis. Ask patient to hold both arms forward, with hands cocked up and fingers spread. Watch for 1 to 2 minutes.

Sudden brief flexions suggest metabolic encephalopathy.

TECHNIQUES	POSSIBLE FINDINGS

Winging of the Scapula. Ask patient to push against the wall of your hand with a partially straightened arm. Inspect scapula. It should stay close to the chest wall.

Winging of scapula away from chest wall suggests weakness of the serratus anterior muscle.

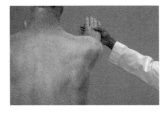
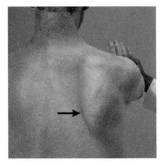

Meningeal Signs. With patient supine, flex head and neck toward chest. Note resistance or pain, and watch for flexion of hips and knees (*Brudzinski's sign*).

Meningeal irritation may cause resistance or pain on flexion during both maneuvers.

Flex one of patient's legs at hip and knee, then straighten knee. Note resistance or pain (*Kernig's sign*).

A compressed lumbosacral nerve root also causes pain on straightening the knee of a raised leg.

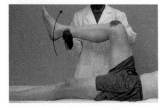

TECHNIQUES	POSSIBLE FINDINGS
○⊸ **Anal Reflex.** With a dull object, stroke outward from anus in four quadrants. Watch for anal contraction.	Loss of reflex suggests lesion at S 2-3-4 level.
○— **Assess the Stuporous or Comatose Patient. Assess** ABCs (airway, breathing, and circulation).	
Take pulse, blood pressure, and rectal temperature.	
Establish level of consciousness with escalating stimuli.	Lethargy, obtundation, stupor, coma

Levels of Consciousness

Alertness	Patient is awake and aware of self and environment. When spoken to in a normal voice, patient looks at you and responds fully and appropriately to stimuli.
Lethargy	When spoken to in a loud voice, patient appears drowsy but opens eyes and looks at you, responds to questions, then falls asleep.
Obtundation	When shaken gently, patient opens eyes and looks at you but responds slowly and is somewhat confused. Alertness and interest in environment are decreased.
Stupor	Patient arouses from sleep only after painful stimuli. Verbal responses are slow or absent. Patient lapses into unresponsiveness when stimulus stops. Patient has minimal awareness of self or environment.
Coma	Despite repeated painful stimuli, patient remains unarousable with eyes closed. No evident response to inner need or external stimuli is shown.

TECHNIQUES	POSSIBLE FINDINGS

Don't dilate pupils, and **don't flex** patient's neck if cervical cord may have been injured.

Observe

- Breathing pattern

Cheyne-Stokes, ataxic breathing

- Pupils

- Ocular movements

Deviation to one side

Note posture of body.

Decorticate rigidity, decerebrate rigidity, flaccid hemiplegia

Check for the *oculocephalic reflex (doll's eye movements)*. Holding upper eyelids open, turn head quickly to each side, then flex and extend patient's neck. This patient's head will be turned to her right.

In a comatose patient with an intact brainstem, the eyes move in the opposite direction, in this case to her left (doll's eye movements). Very deep coma or a lesion in midbrain or pons abolishes this reflex.

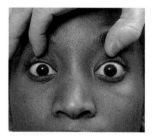 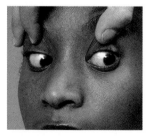

Test for flaccid paralysis.

- Hold forearms vertically; note wrist positions.

A flaccid hand droops to the horizontal.

- From 12 to 18 inches above bed, drop each arm.

A flaccid arm drops more rapidly.

TECHNIQUES	POSSIBLE FINDINGS

- Support both knees in a somewhat flexed position, and then extend each knee and let lower leg drop to the bed.

The flaccid leg drops more rapidly.

- From a similar starting position, release both legs.

A flaccid leg falls into extension and external rotation.

Complete the neurologic and general physical examination.

Recording the Physical Examination— The Nervous System

"*Mental Status:* Alert, relaxed, and cooperative. Thought process coherent. Oriented to person, place, and time. Detailed cognitive testing deferred. *Cranial Nerves:* I—not tested; II through XII intact. *Motor:* Good muscle bulk and tone. Strength 5/5 throughout. Cerebellar: Rapid alternating movements (RAMs), finger-to-nose (F→N), heel-to-shin (H→S) intact. Gait with normal base. Romberg—maintains balance with eyes closed. No pronator drift. *Sensory:* Pinprick, light touch, position, and vibration intact. *Reflexes:* 2+ and symmetric with plantar reflexes downgoing."

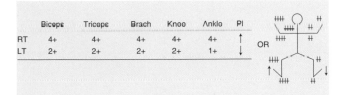

	Biceps	Triceps	Brach	Knee	Ankle	Pl
RT	4+	4+	4+	4+	4+	↑
LT	2+	2+	2+	2+	1+	↓

AIDS TO INTERPRETATION

TABLE 16-1 ■ Disorders of Speech

Aphonia/Dysphonia	A loss (aphonia) or impairment (dysphonia) of voice from disease of larynx or its nerve supply; affects volume, quality, and pitch of voice, as in hoarseness, whisper
Dysarthria	Defective muscular control of lips, tongue, palate, or pharynx, causing nasal, slurred, or indistinct speech; symbolic aspect of language remains intact; caused by motor lesions in central or peripheral nervous system, parkinsonism, or cerebellar disease
Aphasia	A disorder in producing or understanding language, often from lesions in the dominant cerebral hemisphere; two common types: *Wernicke's*—fluent; often rapid, voluble, effortless; inflection and articulation good, but sentences lack meaning and words are malformed or invented *Broca's*—nonfluent, slow, effortful, with few words; inflection and articulation impaired, but words meaningful with nouns, transitive verbs, important adjectives

TABLE 16-2 ■ Delirium and Dementia

	Delirium	Dementia
Timing	Acute onset, fluctuating course, lasts hours/weeks	Insidious onset, slowly progressive, lasts months, years
Sleep pattern	Sleep/wake cycle disrupted	Sleep fragmented
Medical illness or drug toxicity	One or both present	Often absent, especially in Alzheimer's disease
Level of consciousness	Disturbed; decreased awareness, attention	Usually normal until late in course
Activity	Often abnormally decreased or increased	Normal to slow, may be inappropriate
Speech	May be slow, hesitant, fast, incoherent	May be aphasic, show difficulty in finding words
Mood	Labile, may be irritable, fearful, depressed	Often flat, depressed
Thought processes	Disorganized, may be incoherent	Impoverished, with little information
Thought content	Delusions common, often transient	Delusions possible
Perceptions	Illusions, hallucinations	Hallucinations possible
Orientation	Usually disoriented, especially for time. A known place may seem unfamiliar.	Fairly well maintained, but impaired late in course of illness

TABLE 16-3 ■ Facial Paralysis

	Lesion of Peripheral Nervous System	Lesion of Central Nervous System
Side of face affected	Same side as the lesion	Side opposite the lesion
Lower face, e.g., smiling, showing teeth	Weak or paralyzed	Weak or paralyzed
Upper face, e.g., raising eyebrows, wrinkling fore-head, closing eyes	Weak or paralyzed	Normal or slightly weak
Common cause	Bell's palsy (injury to CN VII)	Cerebrovascular accident

TABLE 16-4 ■ Motor Disorders	Peripheral Nervous System Disorder	Central Nervous System Disorder*	Parkinsonism (Basal Ganglia Disorder)	Cerebellar Disorder
Involuntary movements	Often fasciculations	No fasciculations	Resting tremors	Intention tremors
Muscle bulk	Atrophy	Normal or mild atrophy (disuse)	Normal	Normal
Muscle tone	Decreased or absent	Increased, spastic	Increased, rigid	Decreased
Muscle strength	Decreased or lost	Decreased or lost	Normal or slightly decreased	Normal or slightly decreased
Coordination	Unimpaired, though limited by weakness	Slowed and limited by weakness	Good, though slowed and often tremulous	Impaired, ataxic
Reflexes				
Deep tendon	Decreased or absent	Increased	Normal or decreased	Normal or decreased
Plantar	Flexor or absent	Extensor	Flexor	Flexor
Abdominals	Absent	Absent	Normal	Normal

*Upper motor neuron

TABLE 16-5 ■ Involuntary Movements

Tremors. Rhythmic oscillations that may be most evident (1) on movement (intention), (2) at rest, or (3) when maintaining a posture

Intention Tremors   **Resting Tremors**

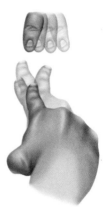

Postural Tremors

Fasciculations. Fine, rapid
flickering of muscle bundles

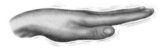

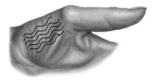

Chorea. Brief, rapid, irregular,
jerky; face, head, arms,
or hands

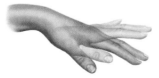

(table continues next page)

TABLE 16-5 ■ Involuntary Movements *(Continued)*

Athetosis. Slow, twisting, writhing; face, distal limbs

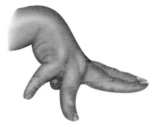

Dystonia. Grotesque, twisted postures, often in trunk or, as shown, in neck (*spasmodic torticollis*)

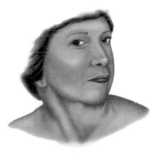

Tics. Brief, irregular, repetitive, coordinated movements, e.g., winking, shrugging

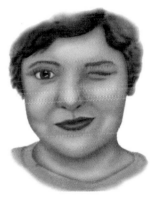

Oral–facial dyskinesias. Rhythmic, repetitive, bizarre movements of face, mouth

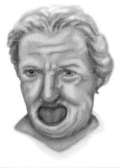

TABLE 16-6 ■ Disorders of Muscle Tone

	Spasticity	Rigidity	Flaccidity	Paratonia
Location of Lesion	Upper motor neuron of the corticospinal tract at any point from the cortex to the spinal cord	Basal ganglia system	Lower motor neuron at any point from the anterior horn cell to the peripheral nerves	Both hemispheres, usually in the frontal lobes
Description	Increased muscle tone (*hypertonia*) that is rate-dependent. Tone is greater when passive movement is rapid, and less when passive movement is slow. Tone is also greater at the extremes of the	Increased resistance that persists throughout the movement arc, independent of rate of movement, is called *lead-pipe rigidity*. With flexion and extension of the	Loss of muscle tone (*hypotonia*), causing the limb to be loose or floppy. The affected limbs may be hyperextensible or even flail-like.	Sudden changes in tone with passive range of motion. Sudden loss of tone that increases the ease of motion is called *mitgehen* (moving with). Sudden increase

movement arc. During rapid passive movement, initial hypertonia may give way suddenly as the limb relaxes. This spastic "catch" and relaxation is known as "clasp-knife" resistance.

wrist or forearm, a superimposed rachetlike jerkiness is called *cogwheel rigidity*.

in tone making motion more difficult is called *gegenhalten* (holding against).

Common Cause		
Stroke, especially late or chronic stage	Parkinsonism	Dementia
Guillain–Barré syndrome; also initial phase of spinal cord injury (spinal shock) or stroke		

TABLE 16-7 ■ Dermatomes

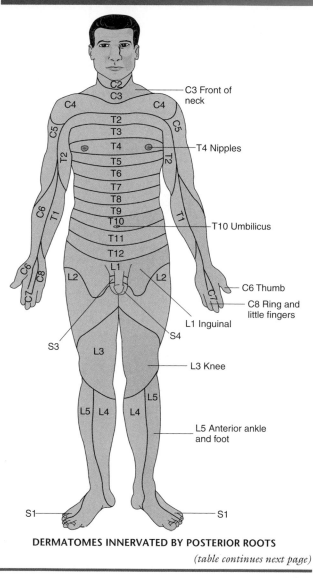

C3 Front of neck

T4 Nipples

T10 Umbilicus

C6 Thumb

C8 Ring and little fingers

L1 Inguinal

L3 Knee

L5 Anterior ankle and foot

DERMATOMES INNERVATED BY POSTERIOR ROOTS

(table continues next page)

TABLE 16-7 ■ Dermatomes (Continued)

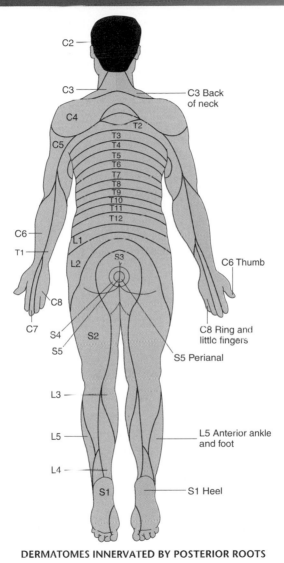

DERMATOMES INNERVATED BY POSTERIOR ROOTS

TABLE 16-8 ■ Pupils in Comatose Patients

Pupillary size, equality, and light reactions help in assessing the cause of coma and in determining the region of the brain that is impaired. Remember that unrelated pupillary abnormalities, including miotic drops for glaucoma or mydriatic drops for a better view of the ocular fundi, may have preceded the coma.

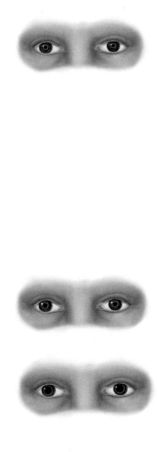

Small or Pinpoint Pupils

Bilaterally small pupils (1–2.5 mm) suggest (1) damage to the sympathetic pathways in the hypothalamus, or (2) metabolic encephalopathy (a diffuse failure of cerebral function that has many causes, including drugs). Light reactions are usually normal.

Pinpoint pupils (<1 mm) suggest (1) a hemorrhage in the pons, or (2) the effects of morphine, heroin, or other narcotics. The light reactions may be seen with a magnifying glass.

Midposition Fixed Pupils

Pupils that are in the *midposition* or *slightly dilated* (4–6 mm) and are *fixed to light* suggest structural damage in the midbrain.

Large Pupils

Bilaterally fixed and dilated pupils may be due to severe anoxia and its sympathomimetic effects, as seen after cardiac arrest. They may also result from atropinelike agents, phenothiazines, or tricyclic antidepressants.

(table continues next page)

TABLE 16-8 ■ Pupils in Comatose Patients *(Continued)*

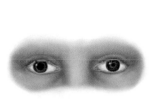

Bilaterally large reactive pupils may be due to cocaine, amphetamine, LSD, or other sympathetic nervous system agonists.

One Large Pupil

A pupil that is *fixed and dilated* warns of herniation of the temporal lobe, causing compression of the oculomotor nerve and midbrain.

Assessing Children: Infancy Through Adolescence

KEY PRINCIPLES OF CHILD DEVELOPMENT

- The first principle is that *child development proceeds along a predictable pathway governed by the maturing brain, marked by developmental milestones.*

- The second principle is that the *range of normal development is wide.* Children mature at different rates.

- The third principle recognizes that *various physical, disease-related, psychological, social, and environmental factors affect child development and health.* For example, chronic diseases and social problems not only can contribute to detectable physical abnormalities but also can influence the rate and course of developmental advancement.

- The fourth principle is that the *child's developmental level affects the nature of the medical history and physical examination.*

THE HEALTH HISTORY

Interviewing Children

- **Establish rapport.** Refer to the infant or child by name. Meet children on their own level. Maintain eye contact at their level (e.g., sit on the floor if needed). Participate in play and talk about their interests.

■ **Work with families.** Ask simple, open-ended questions such as "Are you sick? Tell me about it." followed by more specific questions. Once the parent has started the conversation, direct questions back to the child. Also observe how parents interact with the child.

■ **Identify multiple agendas.** Your job is to discover as many perspectives and agendas as possible.

■ **Use the family as the key resource.** View parents as experts in the care of their child and you as their consultant.

■ **Note hidden agendas.** As with adults, the chief complaint may not relate to the real reason the parent has brought the child to see you.

A Comprehensive Pediatric History

The child's history follows the same outline as the adult's history, with certain *additions* presented here.

Identifying Data. Record date and place of birth, nickname, and first names of parents (and last name of each, if different).

Chief Complaints. Determine if they are the concerns of the child, the parent(s), a schoolteacher, or some other person.

Present Illness. Determine how each family member responds to the child's symptoms, why he or she is concerned, and the secondary gain the illness may provide for the child.

Past History

Birth History. This is especially important when neurologic or developmental problems are present. Get hospital records if necessary.

■ Prenatal—maternal health: medications; tobacco, drug, and alcohol use; vaginal bleeding; weight gain; duration of pregnancy

- Natal—nature of labor and delivery, birth weight, Apgar scores at 1 and 5 minutes

- Neonatal—resuscitation efforts, cyanosis, jaundice, infections, bonding

Feeding History. This is particularly important with undernutrition and overnutrition.

- Breast-feeding—frequency and duration of feeds, difficulties, timing and method of weaning

- Bottle feeding—type; amount; frequency; vomiting; colic; diarrhea; vitamin, iron, and fluoride supplements; introduction of solid foods

- Eating habits—likes and dislikes, types and amounts of food eaten, parental attitudes and responses to feeding problems

Growth and Developmental History. This is important with delayed growth, psychomotor and intellectual retardation, and behavioral disturbances.

- Physical growth—weight, height, and head circumference at birth and less than 10 years; periods of slow or rapid growth

- Developmental milestones—ages child held head up, rolled over, sat, stood, walked, and talked

- Social development—day and night sleeping patterns; toilet training; speech problems; habitual behaviors; discipline problems; school performance; relationships with parents, siblings, and peers

Current Health Status

Allergies. Pay particular attention to childhood allergies: eczema, urticaria, perennial allergic rhinitis, food intolerance, insect hypersensitivity, and recurrent wheezing.

Immunizations. Include dates given and any untoward reactions.

Screening Tests. These are likely to vary according to the child's medical and social conditions. Include those for vision, hearing, cholesterol, tuberculosis, anemia, blood lead, sickle cell disease, and newborn screening results.

HEALTH PROMOTION AND COUNSELING

1. Age-appropriate developmental achievement of the child
   - Physical (maturation, growth, puberty)
   - Motor (gross and fine motor skills)
   - Cognitive (achievement of milestones, language, school performance)
   - Emotional (self-efficacy and mastery, self esteem, independence, morality)
   - Social (social competence, self-responsibility, integration with family and community)

2. Health supervision visits
   - Periodic assessment of medical and oral health, per health supervision schedules (see p. 340)
   - Adjustment of frequency for children or families with special needs

3. Integration of physical examination findings (assure normality, relate findings to healthy lifestyle)

4. Immunizations

5. Screening procedures

6. Anticipatory guidance
   - Healthy habits
   - Nutrition and healthy eating
   - Emotional and mental health
   - Oral health
   - Safety and prevention of injury

- Sexual development and sexuality
- Self-responsibility and efficacy
- Family relationships (interactions, strengths, supports)
- Community interactions (childcare, school)
- Prevention or recognition of illness
- Prevention of risky behaviors and addictions
- School and vocational achievement
- Peer relationships

7. Partnership between health care provider and child, adolescent, and family

TECHNIQUES OF EXAMINATION

■ Sequence of Examination

INFANCY AND EARLY CHILDHOOD

Sequence should vary according to the child's age and comfort level. *Perform nondisturbing maneuvers early and potentially distressing maneuvers toward the end.* For example, palpate the head and neck and auscultate the heart and lungs early; examine the ears and mouth and palpate the abdomen near the end. If the child reports pain in one area, examine that part last.

The format of the pediatric medical record is the same as that of the adult. Thus, although the sequence of the physical examination may vary, convert your written findings back to the traditional format.

LATE CHILDHOOD AND ADOLESCENCE

Use the same sequence as with adults, except examine the most painful areas last.

TECHNIQUES	POSSIBLE FINDINGS

MENTAL AND PHYSICAL STATUS

INFANCY

Observe the parents' affect when talking about the baby; their manner of holding, moving, and dressing the baby; and response to situations that may produce discomfort for the baby. **Observe** a breast or bottle feeding. **Determine** attainment of developmental milestones using the Denver Developmental Screening Test before conducting the physical examination.

Common causes of *developmental delay* include abnormalities in embryonic development, hereditary and genetic disorders, environmental and social problems, other pregnancy or perinatal problems, childhood diseases such as infection (e.g., meningitis), trauma, and severe chronic disease.

EARLY CHILDHOOD

Observe during the interview the degree of sickness or wellness, mood, nutritional state, speech, cry, facial expression, apparent chronologic and emotional age, developmental skills, and parent–child interaction, including separation tolerance, affection, and response to discipline.

LATE CHILDHOOD

Determine orientation to time and place, factual knowledge, and language and number skills. Observe motor skills used in writing, tying laces, buttoning, cutting, and drawing.

TECHNIQUES	**POSSIBLE FINDINGS**

THE GENERAL SURVEY

Measurement of growth is one of the most important indicators of children's health. Deviations from normal may be early indications of an underlying problem. To assess growth, it is important to compare a child's parameters with respect to

Causes of *failure to thrive* can be environmental or psychosocial, or various gastrointestinal, neurologic, cardiac, endocrine, renal, and other diseases.

■ Normal values according to age and sex

■ Prior readings to assess trends

HEIGHT AND WEIGHT

Growth, reflected in increases in height and weight within expected limits, is an excellent indicator of health during infancy and childhood. **Plot** each child's height and weight on standard growth charts to determine progress. See Tables 17-2 to 17-5, pp. 334–337.

Measures above the 97th or below the 3rd percentile, or recent rises or falls from prior levels, require investigation. Reduced growth in height may indicate *endocrine disease,* other *causes of short stature,* or, if weight is also low, other *chronic diseases.*

HEAD CIRCUMFERENCE

Determine head circumference at every physical examination during the first 2 years. See Tables 17-6 and 17-7 on pp. 338–339.

Premature closure of the sutures or *microcephaly* may cause small head size. *Hydrocephalus, subdural hematoma,* or, rarely, *brain tumor* or *inherited syndromes* may cause abnormally large head size.

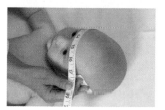

BODY MASS INDEX FOR AGE

Age- and sex-specific charts are now available to assess body mass index (BMI) in children.

Underweight is <5th percentile; at risk of overweight is ≥85th percentile, and overweight is ≥95th percentile.

BLOOD PRESSURE

Hypertension during childhood is more common than previously thought. Recognizing, confirming, and appropriately managing it is important. Blood pressure readings should be part of the physical examination of every child older than 2 years.

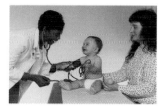

Proper cuff size is essential for accurate determination of blood pressure in children. The most easily used measure of systolic blood pressure in infants and young children is obtained with the *Doppler method.*

The most frequent "cause" of elevated blood pressure in children is probably an *improperly performed examination,* often from an incorrect cuff size.

TECHNIQUES	POSSIBLE FINDINGS

Causes of Sustained Hypertension in Children

Newborn	Middle Childhood
Renal artery disease (stenosis, thrombosis)	Renal parenchymal or arterial disease
Congenital renal malformations	Primary hypertension
Coarctation of the aorta	Coarctation of the aorta

Infancy and Early Childhood	Adolescence
Renal parenchymal or artery disease	Primary hypertension
Coarctation of the aorta	Renal parenchymal disease
	Drug induced

Pulse. The heart rate of children is quite variable.

Tachycardia (>180–200/min) usually indicates *paroxysmal supraventricular tachycardia*. Bradycardia in infants or young children may result from serious underlying disease.

Respiratory Rate. Respiratory rate in infants and children has a greater range and is more responsive to illness, exercise, and emotion than in adults.

Children with respiratory diseases such as *bronchiolitis* or *pneumonia* have rapid respirations (up to 80–90/min), but *also* increased work of breathing.

THE SKIN

Assess

■ *Texture* and *appearance*

Cutis marmorata

■ Vasomotor changes

Acrocyanosis; cyanotic congenital heart disease

TECHNIQUES	POSSIBLE FINDINGS
■ Pigmentation (e.g., Mongolian spots)	*Café-au-lait spots*
■ Hair (e.g., lanugo)	*Midline hair tuft on back*
■ Common skin conditions (e.g., milia, erythema toxicum)	*Herpes simplex*
■ Jaundice	*Hemolytic disease*
■ Turgor	*Dehydration*

THE HEAD

INFANCY

Examine *sutures* and *fontanelles* carefully.

Anterior fontanelle
Posterior fontanelle
Lambdoidal suture
Sagittal suture
Coronal suture
Metopic suture

Check the *face* for symmetry. **Examine** for an overall impression of the *facies;* comparing with the faces of the parents is helpful.

Head small with *microcephaly,* enlarged with *hydrocephaly;* fontanelles full and tense with *meningitis,* closed with *microcephaly,* separated with *increased intracranial pressure* (hydrocephaly, subdural hematoma, and brain tumor)

Swelling from subperiosteal hemorrhage (cephalohematoma) does not cross suture lines; swelling from bleeding associated with a fracture does.

| **TECHNIQUES** | **POSSIBLE FINDINGS** |

PEARLS TO EVALUATE POTENTIALLY ABNORMAL FACIES

Carefully review the history, especially the *family history, pregnancy,* and *perinatal history.*

Note abnormalities, especially of *growth, development,* or *dysmorphic somatic features.*

Measure and plot percentiles, especially of *head circumference, height,* and *weight.*

Consider the three mechanisms of facial dysmorphogenesis:

- Deformations from intrauterine constraint
- Disruptions from amniotic bands or disruption from fetal tissue
- Malformations from an intrinsic abnormality (either face/head or brain)

Examine parents and siblings (similarity may be reassuring or point to a familial disorder).

Determine whether facial features fit a recognizable syndrome. Compare against references, pictures, tables, and databases.

THE NECK

Palpate the *lymph nodes,* and **assess** for any additional masses (e.g., *congenital cysts*).

Lymphadenopathy is usually from viral or bacterial infections. Other neck masses include *malignancy, branchial cleft* or *thyroglossal duct cysts, periauricular cysts and sinuses,* and *nuchal rigidity.*

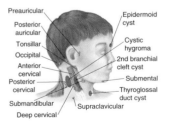

Preauricular
Posterior auricular
Tonsillar
Occipital
Anterior cervical
Posterior cervical
Submandibular
Deep cervical
Epidermoid cyst
Cystic hygroma
2nd branchial cleft cyst
Submental
Thyroglossal duct cyst
Supraclavicular

TECHNIQUES	POSSIBLE FINDINGS

THE EYES

INFANCY

Newborns may look at your face and follow a bright light if you catch them while alert. *Normal visual milestones include:*

Nystagmus, strabismus

Birth	Blinks, may regard face
1 month	Fixes on objects
1½–2 months	Coordinated eye movements
3 months	Eyes converge, baby reaches
12 months	Acuity around 20/50

EARLY CHILDHOOD

The two most important aspects of the eye examination for young children are to test visual acuity in each eye and to determine whether the gaze is conjugate or symmetric.

Strabismus; amblyopia

SPECIAL TECHNIQUE

The corneal light reflex test and the cover-uncover test are particularly useful in young children.

Any difference in visual acuity between eyes is abnormal.

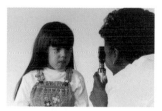

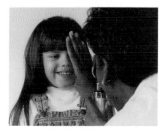

TECHNIQUES	**POSSIBLE FINDINGS**

Age	Visual Acuity
3 months	Eyes converge, baby reaches
12 months	~20/200
Younger than 4 years	20/40
4 years and older	20/30

THE EARS

INFANCY

Check *position,* *shape,* and *features.*

Small, deformed or low-set auricles may indicate associated *congenital defects,* especially renal disease.

Age	Signs That An Infant Can Hear
0–2 months	Startle response and blink to a sudden noise
	Calming down with soothing voice or music
2–3 months	Change in body movements in response to sound
	Change in facial expression to familiar sounds
3–4 months	Turning eyes and head to sound
6–7 months	Turning to listen to voices and conversation

EARLY CHILDHOOD

Examine the ear canal and drum. There are two positions for the child (lying down or sitting), and also two ways to hold the otoscope, as illustrated.

TECHNIQUES

POSSIBLE FINDINGS

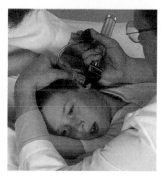

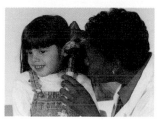

SPECIAL TECHNIQUE

Pneumatic Otoscope. Learn to use a *pneumatic otoscope* to improve your accuracy of diagnosis of otitis media in children.

■ Check for leaks by placing your finger over the tip of the speculum and squeezing the bulb.

■ Insert the speculum, obtaining a proper seal.

Acute otitis media involves a red and bulging tympanic membrane.

■ When air is introduced into the normal ear canal, the tympanic membrane and its light reflex move inward. When air is removed, the tympanic membrane moves outward toward you.

Diminished movement of tympanic membrane with *acute otitis media,* no movement with *otitis media with effusion.* Pain on movement of the pinna with *otitis externa*

TECHNIQUES	POSSIBLE FINDINGS

THE NOSE

INFANCY

Test patency of the nasal passages by alternately occluding each nostril while holding infant's mouth closed.

With *choanal atresia*, the baby cannot breathe if one nostril is occluded.

THE MOUTH AND PHARYNX

INFANCY

For newborns, **inspect** (with a tongue blade and flashlight) and **palpate.**

Supernumerary teeth, Epstein's pearls

You may see a whitish covering on the tongue. If this coating is from milk, you can easily remove it by scraping or wiping it away.

Oral candidiasis (thrush)

EARLY AND LATE CHILDHOOD

For anxious or young children, you may want to leave this examination toward the end. It may require parental restraint.

If you need to use the tongue blade, the best technique is to push down and pull slightly forward toward you while the child says "ahhh." Be careful not to place the blade too far posteriorly, eliciting a gag reflex.

TECHNIQUES	POSSIBLE FINDINGS

Examine the *teeth* for the timing and sequence of eruption, number, character, condition, and position.

Abnormalities of the enamel may reflect local or general disease.

Carefully **inspect** the inside of the upper teeth, as shown.

Nursing bottle caries; dental caries; staining of the teeth, which may be intrinsic or extrinsic

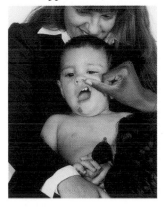

Look for abnormalities of tooth position.

Malocclusion

Note the size, position, symmetry, and appearance of the *tonsils.*

Peritonsillar abscess

THE THORAX AND LUNGS

INFANCY AND EARLY CHILDHOOD

Carefully **assess** respirations and breathing pattern.

Apnea

An important tip is *not* to rush to the stethoscope, but to observe the patient carefully.

Upper respiratory infections may cause nasal flaring.

TECHNIQUES	POSSIBLE FINDINGS

Examination of the Lungs in Infants— Before You Touch the Child!

Assessment	Possible Findings	Explanation
General appearance	Inability to feed or smile Lack of consolability	*Lower respiratory infections* below the vocal cords (e.g., *bronchiolitis, pneumonia*) are common in infants.
Respiratory rate	Tachypnea	
Color	Pallor or cyanosis	
Nasal component of breathing	Nasal flaring (enlargement of both nasal openings during inspiration)	
Audible breath sounds	Grunting (repetitive, short expiratory sound) Wheezing (musical expiratory sound) Stridor (high-pitched, inspiratory noise) Obstruction (lack of breath sounds)	*Acute stridor* is a potentially serious condition with causes such as *laryngotracheobronchitis (croup), epiglottitis, bacterial tracheitis, foreign body, vascular ring*
Work of breathing	Nasal flaring (see above) Grunting (see above) Retractions (or chest indrawing): Supraclavicular (soft tissue above clavicles) Intercostal (indrawing of the skin between ribs) Subcostal (just below the costal margin)	In infants, abnormal work of breathing combined with abnormal findings on auscultation is the best finding for ruling in *pneumonia.*

Distinguishing Upper Airway From Lower Airway Sounds

Technique	Upper Airway	Lower Airway
Compare sounds from nose/stethoscope	Same sounds	Often different sounds
Listen to harshness of sounds	Often harsh and loud	Variable
Note symmetry (left/right)	Symmetric	Often asymmetric
Compare sounds at different locations (higher or lower)	Sounds get louder as stethoscope is moved up on the chest	Sounds often louder lower in chest
Inspiratory vs. expiratory	Almost always inspiratory	Often has expiratory phase

THE HEART

INFANCY

Inspection. **Observe** carefully for any cyanosis.

At birth: *Transposition of the great arteries; pulmonary valve atresia of stenosis*

Within a few days of birth: The above; also *total anomalous pulmonary venous return, hypoplastic left heart syndrome*

Weeks, months, or years of life: The above; also *pulmonary vascular disease with atrial, ventricular, or great vessel shunting*

Palpation. **Palpate** the *peripheral pulses*. The *point of maximal impulse (PMI)* is

No or diminished femoral pulses suggest *coarctation of the aorta*. Weak or thready,

TECHNIQUES	POSSIBLE FINDINGS

not always palpable in infants. *Thrills* are palpable when enough turbulence is within the heart or great vessels.

difficult-to-feel, pulses may reflect *myocardial dysfunction* and *congestive heart failure*.

Auscultation. *Heart rhythm* is evaluated more easily in infants by listening to the heart than by feeling the peripheral pulses.

The most common dysrhythmia in children is *paroxysmal supraventricular tachycardia*.

Heart Sounds. Evaluate S_1 and S_2 carefully. They are normally crisp.

A louder-than-normal pulmonic component, particularly louder than the aortic sound, suggests *pulmonary hypertension*. Persistent splitting of S_2 may indicate a right ventricular volume load, such as *atrial septal defect*.

Heart Murmurs. One of the most challenging aspects to cardiac examination in children is evaluation of *heart murmurs*. In addition to trying to listen to a squirming, perhaps uncooperative child, a major challenge is to distinguish common benign murmurs from unusual or pathologic ones. Most children (indeed, some say nearly all) will have one or more *functional*, or *benign, heart murmurs* before adulthood.

See Table 17-10, Characteristics of Pathologic Heart Murmurs, pp. 342–343.

TECHNIQUES	POSSIBLE FINDINGS

Location of Benign Heart Murmurs in Children

- Venous hum
- Closing ductus
- Carotid bruit
- Pulmonary flow
- Still's

THE BREASTS

LATE CHILDHOOD AND ADOLESCENCE

The most important issue in older children involves assessment of normal maturational development.

See Table 17-11, Sex Maturity Ratings in Girls: Breasts, p. 341.

THE ABDOMEN

INFANCY

Inspect the newborn's *umbilical cord* to detect abnormalities. Normally, there are two thick-walled umbilical arteries and one larger but thin-walled umbilical vein, which is usually located at the 12 o'clock position.

A *single umbilical artery* may be associated with congenital anomalies. *Umbilical hernias* in infants are from a defect in the abdominal wall.

You will find it easy to **palpate** an infant's abdomen because he or she likes being touched.

Abnormal abdominal masses can be associated with kidney, bladder, or bowel tumors. In *pyloric stenosis,* deep palpation in the right

TECHNIQUES	POSSIBLE FINDINGS

upper quadrant or midline can reveal an "olive," or a 2-cm firm pyloric mass.

EARLY AND LATE CHILDHOOD AND ADOLESCENCE

Most children are ticklish when you first place your hand on their abdomens for **palpation.** This reaction tends to disappear, particularly if you distract the child.

A pathologically enlarged liver in children usually is palpable more than 2 cm below the costal margin, has a round, firm edge, and is often tender.

MALE GENITALIA

INFANCY

Inspect with the infant supine.

In 3% of newborns, one or both testes cannot be felt in the scrotum or inguinal canal.

Newborns with _undescended testicles (cryptorchidism);_ in newborns, common scrotal masses are _hydroceles_ and _inguinal hernias_

EARLY AND LATE CHILDHOOD

There is an art to **palpation** of the young boy's scrotum and testes, because many have an extremely active cremasteric reflex that may cause the testes to retract upward into the inguinal canal and thereby appear undescended. A useful technique is to have the boy sit cross-legged on the examining table.

In _precocious puberty,_ the penis and testes are enlarged, with signs of pubertal changes.

A painful testicle requires rapid treatment. _Inguinal hernias_ in older boys present as they do in adult men.

TECHNIQUES	POSSIBLE FINDINGS

ADOLESCENCE

An important goal when examining the adolescent male is to assign a sexual maturity rating.

See Table 17-12, Sex Maturity Ratings in Boys, pp. 345–346.

FEMALE GENITALIA

INFANCY

In the newborn female, genitalia are prominent from the effects of maternal estrogen.

Ambiguous genitalia involves masculinization of the female external genitalia.

EARLY AND LATE CHILDHOOD

For the genital examination, use a calm, gentle approach, including a developmentally appropriate explanation.

Examine the genitalia in an efficient and systematic manner. The normal hymen in infants and young children can have various configurations.

Vaginal discharge in early childhood can result from *perineal irritation* (e.g., bubble baths, soaps), *foreign body, vaginitis,* or *sexually transmitted diseases* from sexual abuse. *Vaginal bleeding* is always concerning. *Abrasions* or signs of trauma to the external genitalia can result from *sexual abuse.*

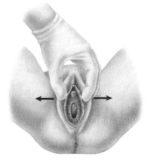

| TECHNIQUES | POSSIBLE FINDINGS |

PHYSICAL SIGNS THAT MAY INDICATE SEXUAL ABUSE IN CHILDREN*

1. Marked and immediate dilatation of the anus in knee–chest position, with no constipation, stool in the vault, or neurologic disorders
2. Hymenal notch or cleft that extends greater than 50% of the inferior hymenal rim (confirmed in knee–chest position)
3. Condyloma acuminata in a child older than 3 years
4. Bruising, abrasions, lacerations, or bite marks of labia or perihymenal tissue
5. Herpes of the anogenital area beyond the neonatal period
6. Purulent or malodorous vaginal discharge in a young girl (all discharges should be cultured and viewed under a microscope for evidence of a sexually transmitted disease)

PHYSICAL SIGNS THAT STRONGLY SUGGEST SEXUAL ABUSE IN CHILDREN*

1. Lacerations, ecchymoses, and newly healed scars of the hymen or the posterior fourchette
2. No hymenal tissue from 3 to 9 o'clock (confirmed in various positions)
3. Healed hymenal transections, especially between 3 and 9 o'clock (complete cleft)
4. Perianal lacerations extending to external sphincter

A sexual-abuse expert must evaluate a child with concerning physical signs for a complete history and sexual abuse examination.

*Any physical sign must be evaluated in light of the entire history, other parts of the physical examination, and laboratory data.

TECHNIQUES	POSSIBLE FINDINGS

ADOLESCENCE

Assign a sexual maturity rating to every female, regardless of chronologic age.

See Table 17-13, Sex Maturity Ratings in Girls: Pubic Hair, p. 347.

THE MUSCULOSKELETAL SYSTEM

INFANCY

The focus is detecting congenital abnormalities, particularly in the hands, spine, hips, legs, and feet.

Skin tags, remnants of digits, polydactyly (extra fingers), or *syndactyly* (webbed fingers) are congenital defects. *Fracture of the clavicle* can occur during a difficult delivery.

Examine the *hips* carefully at each visit for signs of dislocation. There are two major techniques: one to test for a posteriorly dislocated hip (*Ortolani test*), and the other to test for the ability to sublux or dislocate an intact but unstable hip (*Barlow test*).

Ortolani Test

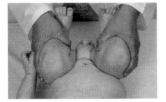

With a *hip dysplasia*, you feel a "clunk."

TECHNIQUES	POSSIBLE FINDINGS

Barlow Test

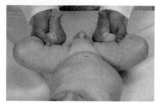

Most newborns are *bowlegged*, reflecting their curled up intrauterine position.

Some normal infants exhibit twisting or *torsion of the tibia* inwardly or outwardly on its longitudinal axis.	Pathologic tibial torsion occurs only in association with *deformities of the feet or hips*.

EARLY AND LATE CHILDHOOD

In older children, abnormalities of the upper extremities are rare in the absence of injury. Observe the child standing and walking barefoot. You also can ask the child to touch the toes, rise from sitting, run a short distance, and pick up objects. You will detect most abnormalities by watching carefully.

TECHNIQUES	POSSIBLE FINDINGS

SPECIAL TECHNIQUE

Testing for Scoliosis. Inspect any child who can stand for *scoliosis*. Make sure the child bends forward with the knees straight (*Adams bend test*). Evaluate any asymmetry in positioning or gait. If you detect scoliosis, use a *scoliometer* to test for the degree.

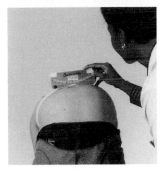

THE NERVOUS SYSTEM

INFANCY

The neurologic screening examination of all newborns should include assessment of mental status, gross and fine motor function, tone, cry, deep tendon reflexes, and primitive reflexes.

Signs of severe neurologic disease include *extreme irritability; persistent asymmetry of posture or extension of extremities; constant turning of head to one side; marked extension of head, neck, and extremities (opisthotonus); severe flaccidity; and limited pain response.*

Evaluate the developing central nervous system by assessing *infantile automatisms,* called *primitive reflexes.*

Suspect a *neurologic* or *developmental abnormality* if primitive reflexes are

- Absent at appropriate age
- Present longer than normal
- Asymmetric
- Associated with posturing or twitching

TECHNIQUES	POSSIBLE FINDINGS

Some neurologic abnormalities produce deficits or slow cognitive and social development. Infants with developmental delay may have abnormal findings on neurologic examination because much of it is based on age-specific norms.

EARLY AND LATE CHILDHOOD

Beyond infancy (when the primitive reflexes have disappeared), the neurologic examination includes the components evaluated in adults. Again, combine the neurologic and developmental assessments. You will need to turn this into a game with the child. The goal is to assess optimal development and neurologic performance, which requires the child's cooperation.

Children with *spastic diplegias* will often have hypotonia as infants.

AIDS TO INTERPRETATION

TABLE 17-1 ■ Classification of a Newborn Infant's Level of Maturity

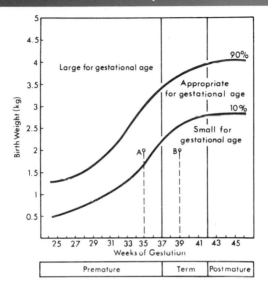

Weight Small for Gestational Age (SGA) = Birth weight <10th percentile on the intrauterine growth curve

Weight Appropriate for Gestational Age (AGA) = Birth weight within the 10th and 90th percentiles on the intrauterine growth curve

Weight Large for Gestational Age (LGA) = Birth weight >90th percentile on the intrauterine growth curve

---

Level of intrauterine growth based on birth weight and gestational age of liveborn, single, white infants. Point A represents a premature infant, while point B indicates an infant of similar birth weight who is mature but small for gestational age; the growth curves are representative of the 10th and 90th percentiles for all of the newborns in the sampling.

Classification of the low-birth-weight infant. In Klaus MH, Fanaroff AA: Care of the High-Rise Neonate, 3rd ed. Philadelphia, WB Saunders, 1986.

TABLE 17-2 ■ Length and Weight Grids for Girls: Birth to 36 Months

Birth to 36 months: Girls
Length-for-age and Weight-for-age percentiles

NAME _____

RECORD # _____

Revised April 20, 2001.
SOURCE: Developed by the National Center for Health Statistics in collaboration with
the National Center for Chronic Disease Prevention and Health Promotion (2000).
http://www.cdc.gov/growthcharts

TABLE 17-3 ■ Stature and Weight Grids for Girls: 2 to 20 Years

2 to 20 years: Girls
Stature-for-age and Weight-for-age percentiles

NAME _____

RECORD # _____

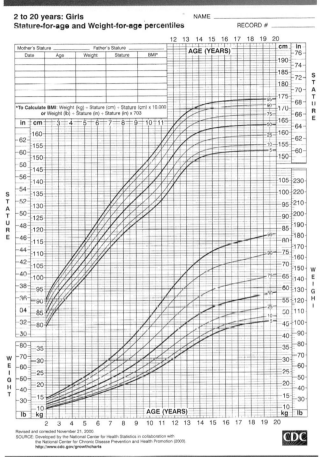

Revised and corrected November 21, 2000.
SOURCE: Developed by the National Center for Health Statistics in collaboration with
the National Center for Chronic Disease Prevention and Health Promotion (2000).
http://www.cdc.gov/growthcharts

TABLE 17-4 ■ Length and Weight Grids for Boys: Birth to 36 Months

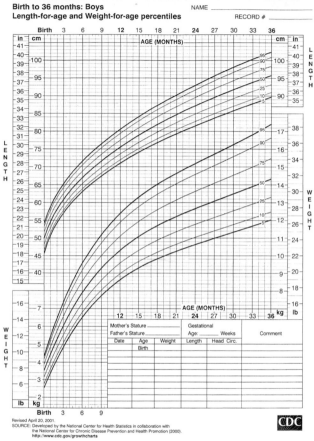

Birth to 36 months: Boys
Length-for-age and Weight-for-age percentiles

NAME _____

RECORD # _____

Revised April 20, 2001.
SOURCE: Developed by the National Center for Health Statistics in collaboration with
the National Center for Chronic Disease Prevention and Health Promotion (2000).
http://www.cdc.gov/growthcharts

CDC

TABLE 17-5 ■ Stature and Weight Grids for Boys: 2 to 20 Years

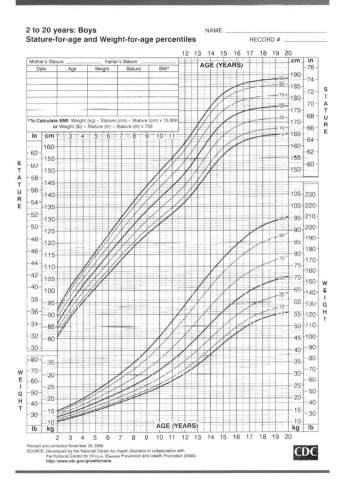

2 to 20 years: Boys
Stature-for-age and Weight-for-age percentiles

TABLE 17-6 ■ Head Circumference and Weight Grids for Girls: Birth to 36 Months

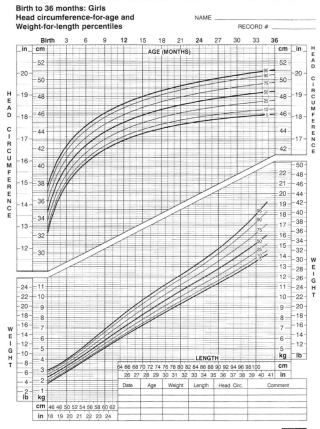

Birth to 36 months: Girls
Head circumference-for-age and
Weight-for-length percentiles

NAME _____

RECORD # _____

SOURCE: Developed by the National Center for Health Statistics in collaboration with the National Center for Chronic Disease Prevention and Health Promotion (2000). http://www.cdc.gov/growthcharts

TABLE 17-7 ■ Head Circumference and Weight Grids for Boys: Birth to 36 Months

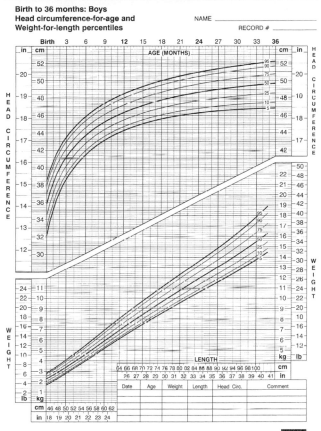

Birth to 36 months: Boys
Head circumference-for-age and
Weight-for-length percentiles

NAME _____

RECORD # _____

SOURCE: Developed by the National Center for Health Statistics in collaboration with the National Center for Chronic Disease Prevention and Health Promotion (2000). http://www.cdc.gov/growthcharts

TABLE 17-8 ■ Recommendations for Preventive Pediatric Health Care

Each child and family is unique; therefore, these recommendation are designed for the care of children who are receiving competent parenting, have no manifestation of any important health problems, and are growing and developing in satisfactory fashion. Additional visits may become necessary if circumstances suggest variation from normal.

AGE	2-4 days[1]	By 1 mo	2 mo	4 mo	6 mo	8 mo	10 mo	12 mo	15 mo	18 mo	24 mo	3 y	4 y	5 y	6 y	8 y	10 y	11 y	12 y	13 y	14 y	15 y	16 y	17 y	18 y	19 y	20 y+
	INFANCY											**EARLY CHILDHOOD**		**MIDDLE CHILDHOOD**					**ADOLESCENCE**								
HISTORY Initial / Interval	•	•	•	•	•	•	•	•	•	•	•	•	•	•	•	•	•	•	•	•	•	•	•	•	•	•	•
MEASUREMENTS Height and Weight	•	•	•	•	•	•	•	•	•	•	•	•	•	•	•	•	•	•	•	•	•	•	•	•	•	•	•
Head Circumference	•	•	•	•	•	•	•	•	•	•																	
Blood Pressure												•	•	•	•	•	•	•	•	•	•	•	•	•	•	•	•
SENSORY SCREENING Vision	S	S	S	S	S	S	S	S	S	S	S	O	O	O	O	O	O	S	O	S	S	O	S	S	O	S	S
Hearing	S	S	S	S	S	S	S	S	S	S	S	S	S	O	O	O	O	S	O	S	S	O	S	S	O	S	S
DEVELOPMENTAL/ BEHAVIORAL ASSESSMENT[2]	•	•	•	•	•	•	•	•	•	•	•	•	•	•	•	•	•	•	•	•	•	•	•	•	•	•	•
PHYSICAL EXAMINATION[3]	•	•	•	•	•	•	•	•	•	•	•	•	•	•	•	•	•	•	•	•	•	•	•	•	•	•	•

1. For newborns discharged in less than 48 hours after delivery
2. By history and appropriate physical examination; if suspicious, by specific objective development testing
3. At each visit, a complete physical examination is essential, with infant totally unclothed, older child undressed and suitably draped

Key • = to be performed   S = subjective, by history
     O = objective, by a standard testing method

Adapted from Recommendations for Preventive Pediatric Health Care promulgated by the American Academy of Pediatrics Committee on Practice and Ambulatory Medicine. Pediatrics 96:373, 1995. Additional recommendations made by the Committee regarding screening for metabolic disorders, tuberculosis, anemia, and urinary tract diseases, administration of immunizations, provision of anticipatory guidance, and initial dental referral are not included in the above summation.

TABLE 17-9 ■ Hypertension in Childhood

Hypertension can start in childhood. While young children with elevated blood pressure are more likely to have a renal, cardiac, or endocrine cause, adolescents with hypertension are most likely to have primary or essential hypertension.

This child developed hypertension during adolescence, and it "tracked" into adulthood. Children tend to remain in the same percentile for blood pressure as they grow. This tracking of blood pressure continues into adulthood, supporting the concept that adult essential hypertension begins during childhood.

The consequences of untreated hypertension can be severe.

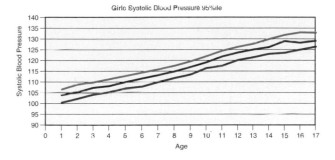

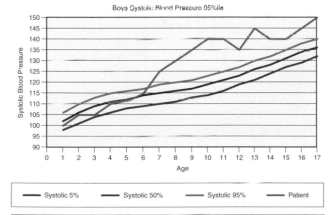

TABLE 17-10 ■ Characteristics of Pathologic
Heart Murmurs

Congenital Defect	Characteristics of Murmur
Pulmonary Valve Stenosis *Mild* 	*Location.* Upper left sternal border *Radiation.* In mild degrees of stenosis, the murmur may be heard over the course of the pulmonary arteries in the lung fields.
Moderate 	*Intensity.* Increases in intensity and duration as the degree of obstruction increases *Quality.* Ejection, peaking later in systole as the obstruction increases
Severe 	
Aortic Valve Stenosis 	*Location.* Midsternum, upper right sternal border *Radiation.* To the carotid arteries and suprasternal notch; may also be a thrill *Intensity.* Varies, louder with increasingly severe obstruction *Quality.* An ejection, often harsh, systolic murmur
Tetralogy of Fallot *With pulmonic stenosis* 	*General.* Variable cyanosis, increasing with activity *Location.* Mid-to-upper left sternal border. If pulmonary atresia, there is no systolic murmur but the continuous murmur of ductus arteriosus flow at upper left sternal border or in the back.

(table continues next page)

TABLE 17-10 ■ Characteristics of Pathologic Heart Murmurs *(Continued)*

Congenital Defect	Characteristics of Murmur
With pulmonic atresia 	*Radiation.* Little, to upper left sternal border, occasionally to lung fields *Intensity.* Usually Grade III–IV *Quality.* Midpeaking, systolic ejection murmur
Transposition of the Great Arteries	*General.* Intense generalized cyanosis *Location.* No characteristic murmur. If a murmur is present, it may reflect an associated defect such as VSD or patent ductus arteriosus. *Radiation.* Depends on associated abnormalities *Quality.* Depends on associated abnormalities
Ventricular Septal Defect *Small to moderate* 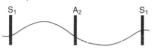	*Location.* Lower left sternal border *Radiation.* Little *Intensity.* Variable, only partially determined by the size of the shunt. Small shunts with a high pressure gradient may have very loud murmurs. Large defects with elevated pulmonary vascular resistance may have no murmur. Grade II–IV/VI with a thrill if Grade IV/VI or higher.

TABLE 17-11 ■ Sex Maturity Ratings in Girls: Breasts

Stage 1

Preadolescent—elevation of nipple only

Stage 2   Stage 3

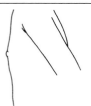   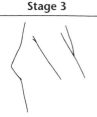

Breast bud stage. Elevation of   Further enlargement and
breast and nipple as a small   elevation of breast and
mound; enlargement of   areola, with no separation
areolar diameter   of the contours

Stage 4   Stage 5

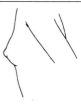   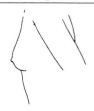

Projection of areola and nipple   Mature stage; projection of
to form a secondary mound   nipple only. Areola has
above the level of the breast   receded to general contour
                                        of the breast (although in
                                        some normal individuals
                                        areola continues to form a
                                        secondary mound).

(Illustrations through the courtesy of W. A. Daniel, Jr.)

TABLE 17-12 ■ Sex Maturity

In assigning SMRs in boys, observe each of the three characteristics separately. Record two separate ratings: pubic hair and genital. If the penis and testes differ in their stages, average the two into a single figure for the genital rating

	Pubic Hair	Genitalia	
		Penis	Testes and Scrotum
Stage 1	Preadolescent—no pubic hair except for the fine body hair (vellus hair) similar to that on the abdomen	Preadolescent—same size and proportions as in childhood	Preadolescent—same size and proportions as in childhood
Stage 2	Sparse growth of long, slightly pigmented, downy hair, straight or only slightly curled, chiefly at the base of the penis	Slight to no enlargement	Testes larger; scrotum larger, somewhat reddened, and altered in texture
Stage 3	Darker, coarser, curlier hair spreading sparsely over the pubic symphysis	Larger, especially in length	Further enlarged

(table continues next page)

TABLE 17-12 ■ Sex Maturity (Continued)

	Pubic Hair	Genitalia	
		Penis	Testes and Scrotum
Stage 4	Coarse and curly hair, as in the adult; area covered greater than in stage 3 but not as great as in the adult and not yet including the thighs	Further enlarged in length and breadth, with development of the glans	Further enlarged; scrotal skin darkened
Stage 5	Hair adult quantity and quality, spread to the medial surfaces of the thighs but not up over the abdomen	Adult in size and shape	Adult in size and shape

(Illustrations through the courtesy of W. A. Daniel, Jr.)

TABLE 17-13 ■ Sex Maturity Ratings in Girls: Pubic Hair

Stage 1 — Preadolescent—no pubic hair except for the fine body hair (vellus hair) similar to that on the abdomen

Stage 2 — Sparse growth of long, slightly pigmented, downy hair, straight or only slightly curled, chiefly along the labia

Stage 3 — Darker, coarser, curlier hair, spreading sparsely over the pubic symphysis

Stage 4 — Coarse and curly hair as in adults; area covered greater than in stage 3 but not as great as in the adult and not yet including the thighs

Stage 5 — Hair adult in quantity and quality, spread on the medial surfaces of the thighs but not up over the abdomen

(Illustrations through the courtesy of W. A. Daniel, Jr.)

Clinical Reasoning, Assessment, and Plan

■ Assessment and Plan: The Process of Clinical Reasoning

Because assessment takes place in the clinician's mind, the process of clinical reasoning often seems inaccessible to beginning students. As an active learner, be sure to ask your teachers and clinicians to elaborate on the fine points of their clinical reasoning and decision making.

As you gain experience, your thinking will begin at the outset of the patient encounter, not at the end. Listed below are principles underlying the process of clinical reasoning and certain explicit steps to help guide your thinking.

IDENTIFYING PROBLEMS AND MAKING DIAGNOSES: STEPS IN CLINICAL REASONING

- **Identify abnormal findings.** Make a list of the patient's *symptoms*, the *signs* you observed during physical examination, and any available results of laboratory reports.
- **Localize these findings anatomically.** The symptom of a scratchy throat and the sign of an erythematous inflamed pharynx, for example, clearly localize the problem to the pharynx. Some symptoms and signs cannot be localized, such as fatigue or fever, but are useful in the next steps.
- **Interpret the findings in terms of the probable process.** There are a number of *pathologic* processes, including congenital, inflammatory or infectious,

(continued)

immunologic, neoplastic, metabolic, nutritional,
degenerative, vascular, traumatic, and toxic. Other
problems are *pathophysiologic,* reflecting derangements of
biologic functions, such as congestive heart failure. Still
other problems are *psychopathologic,* such as headache as
an expression of a somatization disorder.

■ **Make hypotheses about the nature of the patient's
problems.** Draw on your knowledge, experience, and
reading about patterns of abnormalities and diseases. The
following steps should help:

1. Select the most specific and critical findings to support
   your hypothesis.
2. Match your findings against all the conditions you know
   that can produce them.
3. Eliminate the diagnostic possibilities that fail to explain
   the findings.
4. Weigh the competing possibilities and select the most
   likely diagnosis.
5. Give special attention to potentially life-threatening and
   treatable conditions. One rule of thumb is *always to
   include "the worst case scenario"* in your list of differential
   diagnoses and make sure you have ruled out that
   possibility based on your findings and patient assessment.

■ **Test your hypotheses.** You may need further history,
additional maneuvers on physical examination, or
laboratory studies or x-rays to confirm or to rule out your
tentative diagnosis or to clarify which of a few possible
diagnoses is most likely.

■ **Establish a working diagnosis.** Make this at the highest
level of explicitness and certainty that the data allow. You
may be limited to a symptom, such as "tension headache,
cause unknown." At other times, you can define a problem
explicitly in terms of its structure, process, and cause, such
as "bacterial meningitis, pneumococcal." Routinely listing
Health Maintenance helps you track several important health
concerns more effectively: immunizations, screening
measures (e.g., mammograms, prostate examinations),

(continued)

IDENTIFYING PROBLEMS AND MAKING DIAGNOSES: STEPS IN CLINICAL REASONING (Continued)

instructions regarding nutrition and breast or testicular self-examinations, recommendations about exercise or use of seat belts, and responses to important life events.

■ **Develop a plan agreeable to the patient.** Identify and record a *Plan* for each patient problem, ranging from tests to confirm or further evaluate a diagnosis; consultations for subspecialty evaluation; additions, deletions, or changes in medication; or arranging a family meeting.

■ The Case of Mrs. N: Assessment and Plan

Now review the assessment and plan for Mrs. N.

ASSESSMENT AND PLAN FOR MRS. N

1. **Migraine headaches.** 54-year-old woman with migraine headaches since childhood, with a throbbing vascular pattern and frequent nausea and vomiting. Headaches are associated with stress and relieved by sleep and cold compresses. There is no papilledema, and there are no motor or sensory deficits on the neurologic examination. The differential diagnosis includes tension headache, also associated with stress, but there is no relief with massage, and the pain is more throbbing than aching. There are no fever, stiff neck, or focal findings to suggest meningitis, and lifelong recurrent pattern makes subarachnoid hemorrhage unlikely (usually described as "the worst headache of my life").

Plan:

■ Discuss features of migraine vs. tension headaches.
■ Discuss biofeedback and stress management.
■ Advise patient to avoid caffeine, including coffee, colas, and other carbonated beverages.

(continued)

ASSESSMENT AND PLAN FOR MRS. N (Continued)

- Start NSAIDs for headache, as needed.
- If needed next visit, begin prophylactic medication, because patient is having more than three migraines per month.

2. **Elevated blood pressure.** Systolic hypertension with wide cuff is present. May be related to obesity, also to anxiety from first visit. No evidence of end-organ damage to retina or heart.

Plan:

- Discuss standards for assessing blood pressure.
- Recheck blood pressure in 1 month, using wide cuff.
- Review urinalysis.
- Introduce weight reduction and/or exercise programs (see #4).
- Reduce salt intake.

3. **Cystocele with occasional stress incontinence.** Cystocele on pelvic examination, probably related to bladder relaxation. Patient is perimenopausal. Incontinence reported with coughing, suggesting alteration in bladder neck anatomy. No dysuria, fever, flank pain. Not on any contributing medications. Usually involves small amounts of urine, no dribbling, so doubt urge or overflow incontinence.

Plan:

- Explain cause of stress incontinence.
- Review urinalysis.
- Recommend Kegel's exercises.
- Consider topical estrogen cream to vagina next visit if no improvement.

4. **Overweight.** Patient 5'2", weighs 143 lbs. BMI is ~26.

Plan:

- Explore diet history, ask patient to keep food intake diary.
- Explore motivation to lose weight, set target for weight loss by next visit.
- Schedule visit with dietician.

(continued)

ASSESSMENT AND PLAN FOR MRS. N (Continued)

- Discuss exercise program, specifically, walking 30 minutes at least three times a week.

5. **Family stress.** Son-in-law with alcohol problem; daughter and grandchildren seeking refuge in patient's apartment, leading to tensions in these relationships. Patient also has financial constraints. Stress currently situational. No evidence of major depression at present.

Plan:

- Explore patient's views on strategies to cope with sources of stress.
- Explore sources of support, including Al-Anon for daughter and financial counseling for patient.
- Continue to monitor for depression.

6. **Occasional musculoskeletal low back pain.** Usually with prolonged standing. No history of trauma or motor vehicle accident. Pain does not radiate; no tenderness or motor-sensory deficits on examination. Doubt disc or nerve root compression, trochanteric bursitis, sacroillitis.

Plan:

- Review benefits of weight loss and exercises to strengthen low back muscles.

7. **Tobacco abuse.** 1 pack per day for 36 years.

Plan:

- Check peak flow or FEV_1/FVC on office spirometry.
- Give strong warning to stop smoking.
- Offer referral to tobacco cessation program.
- Offer patch, current treatment to enhance abstinence.

8. **Varicose veins, lower extremities.** No complaints currently.
9. **History of right pyelonephritis, 1982.**
10. **Ampicillin allergy.** Developed rash but no other allergic reaction.

(continued)

ASSESSMENT AND PLAN FOR MRS. N (Continued)

11. **Health maintenance.** Last Pap smear 1998; has never had a mammogram.

Plan:

- Teach patient breast self-examination; schedule mammogram.
- Schedule Pap smear next visit.
- Provide three stool guaiac cards; next visit discuss screening flexible sigmoidoscopy.
- Suggest dental care for mild gingivitis.
- Advise patient to move medications and caustic cleaning agents to locked cabinet, if possible, above shoulder height.

■ Approaching the Challenges of Clinical Data

As you can see from the case of Mrs. N, organizing the patient's clinical data poses several challenges. The following guidelines will help you address these challenges.

■ **Clustering data into single versus multiple problems.** The patient's *age* may help. Young people are more likely to have a single disease, while older people tend to have multiple diseases. The *timing* of symptoms is often useful. For example, an episode of pharyngitis 6 weeks ago probably is unrelated to fever, chills, pleuritic chest pain, and cough that prompt an office visit today.

If symptoms and signs are in a single system, one disease may explain them. Problems in different, apparently unrelated systems often require more than one explanation. Again, knowledge of disease patterns is necessary.

Some diseases involve *multisystem conditions.* To explain cough, hemoptysis, and weight loss in a 60-year-old plumber who has smoked cigarettes for 40 years, you probably even now would rank lung cancer high in your list of differential diagnoses.

■ **Sifting through an extensive array of data.** Try to *tease out separate clusters of observations and analyze one cluster at a time.* You also can *ask a series of key questions* that may steer your thinking in one direction. For example, you may ask what produces and relieves the patient's chest pain. If the answer is exercise and rest, you can focus on the cardiovascular and musculoskeletal systems and set the gastrointestinal system aside.

■ **Assessing the quality of the data.** To avoid errors in interpreting clinical information, acquire the habits of skilled clinicians, summarized in the following.

TIPS FOR ENSURING THE QUALITY OF PATIENT DATA

- Ask open-ended questions and listen carefully and patiently to the patient's story.
- Craft a thorough and systematic sequence to history taking and physical examination.
- Keep an open mind toward both the patient and the data.
- Always include "the worst-case scenario" in your list of possible explanations of the patient's problem, and make sure it can be eliminated safely.
- Analyze any mistakes in data collection or interpretation.
- Confer with colleagues and review the pertinent medical literature to clarify uncertainties.
- Apply principles of data analysis to patient information and testing.

■ **Improving your assessment of clinical data and laboratory tests.** Apply several key principles for selecting and using clinical data and tests: *reliability, validity, sensitivity, specificity,* and *predictive value.* Learn to apply these principles to your clinical findings and the tests you order.

■ **Displaying clinical data.** To use these principles, it is important to display the data in the 2 × 2 format diagrammed on page 357. Always using this format will ensure the accuracy of your calculations of sensitivity, specificity, and predictive value.

PRINCIPLES OF TEST SELECTION AND USE

Reliability

Indicates how well repeated measurements of the same relatively stable phenomenon will give the same result, also known as **precision.** Reliability may be measured for one or more observers.

Example: If on several occasions one clinician consistently percusses the same span of a patient's liver dullness, *intraobserver reliability* is good. If, on the other hand, several observers find quite different spans of liver dullness on the same patient, *interobserver reliability* is poor.

Validity

Indicates how closely a given observation agrees with "the true state of affairs," or the best possible measure of reality.

Example: Blood pressure measurements by mercury-based sphygmomanometers are less valid than intra-arterial pressure tracings.

Sensitivity

Identifies the proportion of people who test positive in a group known to have the disease or condition, or the proportion who are *true positives* compared to the total number of people who actually have the disease. When the observation or test is negative in people who have the disease, the result is termed *false negative. Good observations or tests have a sensitivity of more than 90% and help rule out disease because false negatives are few. Such observations or tests are especially useful for screening.*

Example: The sensitivity of Homan's sign in the diagnosis of deep venous thrombosis (DVT) of the calf is 50%. In other words, compared to a group of patients with DVT confirmed by phlebogram, a much better test, only 50% will have a positive Homan's sign, so this sign, if absent, is not helpful, because 50% of patients may have a DVT.

Specificity

Identifies the proportion of people who test negative in a group known to be *without* a given disease or condition, or the proportion of people who are "true negatives" compared to the total number of people without the disease. When the

(continued)

PRINCIPLES OF TEST SELECTION
AND USE (Continued)

observation or test is positive in people without the disease, the result is termed "false positive." Good observations or tests have a specificity of more than 90% and help "rule in" disease, because the test is rarely positive when disease is absent, and false positives are few.

Example: The specificity of serum amylase in patients with possible acute pancreatitis is 70%. In other words, of 100 patients without pancreatitis, 70% will have a normal serum amylase; in 30%, the serum amylase will be falsely elevated.

Predictive Value

Indicates how well a given symptom, sign, or test result— either positive or negative—predicts the presence or absence of disease.

Positive predictive value is the probability of disease in a patient with a positive (abnormal) test, or the proportion of "true positives" out of the total population tested.

Example: In a group of women with palpable breast nodules in a cancer screening program, the proportion with confirmed breast cancer would constitute the *positive predictive value* of palpable breast nodules for diagnosing breast cancer.

Negative predictive value is the probability of not having the condition or disease when the test is negative, or normal, or the proportion of "true negatives" out of the total population tested.

Example: In a group of women without palpable breast nodules in a cancer screening program, the proportion without confirmed breast cancer constitutes the *negative predictive value* of absence of breast nodules.

Validity—the closeness with which a measurement reflects the true value of an object

Reliability—the reproducibility of a measurement

Sensitivity, specificity, and *predictive values* are illustrated in a 2 × 2 table, as shown below in an example of 200 people, half of whom have the disease in question. In this example, the disease prevalence of 50% is much higher than in most clinical situations. Because the positive predictive value increases with prevalence, its calculated value here is accordingly and unrealistically high.

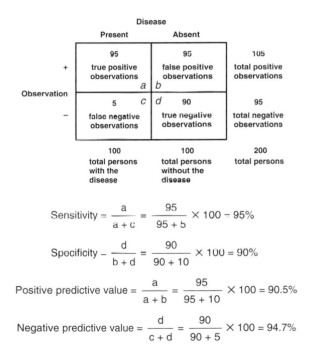

$$\text{Sensitivity} = \frac{a}{a + c} = \frac{95}{95 + 5} \times 100 = 95\%$$

$$\text{Specificity} = \frac{d}{b + d} = \frac{90}{90 + 10} \times 100 = 90\%$$

$$\text{Positive predictive value} = \frac{a}{a + b} = \frac{95}{95 + 10} \times 100 = 90.5\%$$

$$\text{Negative predictive value} = \frac{d}{c + d} = \frac{90}{90 + 5} \times 100 = 94.7\%$$

■ Organizing the Patient Record

A clear, well-organized clinical record is one of the most important adjuncts to your patient care. Think about the *order and readability* of the record and the *amount of detail* needed. Use the following checklist to make sure your record is clear, informative, and easy to follow.

CHECKLIST FOR YOUR PATIENT RECORD

Is the order clear?

Order is imperative. Make sure that future readers, including you, can find specific points of information easily. Keep the *subjective* items of the history, for example, in the history; do not let them stray into the physical examination. Did you . . .

■ Make the headings clear?
■ Accent your organization with indentations and spacing?
■ Arrange the *Present Illness* in chronologic order, starting with the current episode, then filling in relevant background information?

Do the data included contribute directly to the assessment?

Spell out the supporting data—both positive and negative— for every problem or diagnosis that you identify.

Are pertinent negatives specifically described?

Often portions of the history or examination suggest a potential or actual abnormality.

Examples: For the patient with notable bruises, record the "pertinent negatives," such as the absence of injury or violence, familial bleeding disorders, or medications or nutritional deficits that might lead to bruising.

For the patient who is depressed but not suicidal, record both facts. In the patient with a transient mood swing, on the other hand, a comment on suicide is unnecessary.

(continued)

CHECKLIST FOR YOUR PATIENT RECORD (Continued)

Are there overgeneralizations or omissions of important data?

Remember that data not recorded are data lost. No matter how vividly you can recall selected details today, you probably will not remember them in a few months. The phrase "neurologic exam negative," even in your own handwriting, may leave you wondering in a few months' time, "Did I really do the sensory exam?"

Is there too much detail?

Avoid burying important information in a mass of excessive detail, to be discovered by only the most persistent reader. *Omit most negative findings* unless they relate directly to the patient's complaints or to specific exclusions in your diagnostic assessment. *Do not list abnormalities that you did not observe. Instead, concentrate on a few major ones,* such as "no heart murmurs," and try to describe structures concisely and positively.

Examples. "Cervix pink and smooth" indicates you saw no redness, ulcers, nodules, masses, cysts or other suspicious lesions, but the description is shorter and much more readable.

You can omit certain body structures even though you examined them, such as normal eyebrows and eyelashes.

Are phrases and short words used appropriately? Is there unnecessary repetition of data?

Omit unnecessary words, such as those in parentheses in the examples below. This saves valuable time and space.

Examples. "Cervix is pink (in color)." "Lungs are resonant (to percussion)." "Liver is tender (to palpation)." "Both (right and left) ears with cerumen." "II/VI systolic ejection murmur (audible)." "Thorax symmetric (bilaterally)."

Omit repetitive introductory phrases such as "The patient reports no . . . ," because readers assume the patient is the source of the history unless otherwise specified.

Use short words instead of longer, fancier ones when they mean the same thing, such as "felt" for "palpated" or "heard" for "auscultated."

(continued)

<u>CHECKLIST FOR YOUR PATIENT RECORD</u> (Continued)

Describe what you observed, not what you did. "Optic discs seen" is less informative than "disc margins sharp," even if it marks your first glimpse as an examiner!

Is the written style succinct? Is there excessive use of abbreviations?

Records are scientific and legal documents, so they should be clear and understandable. Using words and brief phrases instead of whole sentences is common, but abbreviations and symbols should be used only if they are readily understood. Likewise, an overly elegant style is less appealing than a concise summary.

Be sure your record is legible; otherwise, all that you have recorded is worthless to your readers.

Are diagrams and precise measurements included where appropriate?

Diagrams add greatly to the clarity of the record.

Examples. Study the examples below:

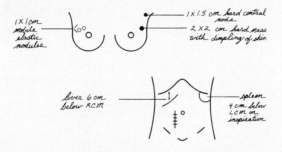

To ensure accurate evaluations and future comparisons, make measurements in centimeters, not in fruits, nuts, or vegetables.

Example. "1 × 1 cm lymph node" vs. "a pea-sized lymph node. . ." Or "2 × 2 cm mass on the left lobe of the prostate" vs. "a walnut-sized prostate mass."

(continued)

CHECKLIST FOR YOUR PATIENT RECORD (Continued)

Is the tone of the write-up neutral and professional?

It is important to be objective. Hostile, moralizing, or disapproving comments have no place in the patient's record. Never use words, penmanship, or punctuation that are inflammatory or demeaning.

Example. Comments such as "Patient DRUNK and LATE TO CLINIC AGAIN!!" are unprofessional and set a bad example for other providers reading the chart. They also might prove difficult to defend in a legal setting.

Once you have completed your assessment and written record, you will find it helpful to generate a *Problem List* that summarizes the patient's problems for the front of the office or hospital chart. A sample *Problem List* for Mrs. N. is provided next.

Sample Problem List		
Date Entered	**Problem No.**	**Problem**
7/15/03	1	Migraine headaches
	2	Elevated blood pressure
	3	Cystocele with occasional stress incontinence
	4	Overweight
	5	Family stress
	6	Low back pain
	7	Tobacco abuse
	8	Varicose veins
	9	History of right pyelonephritis
	10	Allergy to ampicillin
	11	Health maintenance

Index

Note: Page numbers followed by *b* indicates boxed material; those followed by *t* indicates tables.